AF655827

Soulful Serenity: Yoga and Meditation for Blissful Life

Soulful Serenity: Yoga and Meditation for Blissful Life

Dr. Khushboo Gupta, Assistant Professor, Trilok Singh TT College, Lakshmangarh, Sikar, Rajasthan, India

Dr. Gopeswar Mukharjee, Professor, M.B.B.S., D.C.P & amp; M.D. (Path), Ph.D. (Path) Professor & amp; Dean, Brainware University, Kolkata, West Bengal, India

Dr. Sparsha Deep EM, Professor & Head, Department of Pharmacology and Chief Coordinator of Clinical Skills & Simulation Lab at Shridevi Institute of Medical Sciences & Research Hospital (SIMS&RH), Tumakuru, Karnataka.

Dr. Sangeeta, Assistant Professor, Home- Science (Food & Nutrition), Ramabai Govt. Women Post Graduate College- Akbarpur, Ambedkar Nagar- Uttar-Pradesh, India

Dr. Vamshi Krishna Kondle, Vice Principal, Professor & Head of the Department Paediatrics, RVMIMS&RC, Telangana

HEMAKSHEE PUBLICATION

Soulful Serenity: Yoga and Meditation for Blissful Life

Edition: 2024
ISBN (Softback): 978-93-48873-86-6
Copyright © **Publisher**
All Rights Reserved.

This book has been published with all reasonable efforts taken to make the material error-free after the consent of the author. No part of this book shall be used, reproduced in any manner whatsoever without written permission from the editor of the book @ Khushboo Gupta and publisher @ Hemakshee Publication, except in the case of brief quotations embodied in critical articles and reviews.

The Chapter Authors of this book is solely responsible and liable for its content. The Content of this book shall not constitute or be construed or deemed to reflect the opinion or expression of the Publisher or Editor. Neither the Publisher nor Editor endorse or approve the Content of this book or guarantee the reliability, accuracy or completeness of the Content published herein and do not make any representations or warranties of any kind, express or implied, including but not limited to the implied warranties of merchantability, fitness for a particular purpose. The Publisher and Editor shall not be liable whatsoever for any errors, omissions, whether such errors or omissions result from negligence, accident, or any other cause or claims for loss or damages of any kind, including without limitation, indirect or consequential loss or damage arising out of use, inability to use, or about the reliability, accuracy or sufficiency of the information contained in this book. All disputes are subject to the jurisdiction of competent courts to Sikar, Rajasthan, India.

Published by Hemakshee Publication
Printed and Distributed by pothi.com

HEMAKSHEE PUBLICATION

Sikar, Rajasthan, India

Email: support@hemaksheepublication.com

Website: www.hemaksheepublication.com

Contents

Preface

Soulful Serenity: Yoga and Meditation for Blissful Life is a heartfelt exploration of the transformative power of yoga and meditation, aimed at guiding individuals toward a balanced, peaceful, and fulfilled life. This book is not merely a collection of theoretical concepts but a reflection of the collective effort and wisdom shared during a conceptual paper writing event organized on **International Yoga Day, 2024** by **"Jeevan Asheesh Samiti"**, a non-profit organization from Kota city, Rajasthan in collaboration with the YouTube channel **"Dietitian Ki Salah"** (an educational plateform for integrated health, wellness, wholesome nutrition, fitness and food).

The event served as an invaluable platform where experts, practitioners, and wellness enthusiasts gathered to share their knowledge and insights on the practical applications of yoga and meditation in modern life. The chapters in this edited book are the direct result of those discussions, focusing on how yoga and meditation can help individuals manage stress, enhance emotional well-being, and foster a deeper connection with themselves.

Each chapter represents a conceptual exploration into different aspects of yoga, from its role in holistic health and mindful living to its transformative impact during specific life stages, including pregnancy and motherhood. This book brings together the ancient wisdom of yoga with the latest research and evidence-based findings, creating a resource that is both accessible and deeply rooted in tradition.

The contributions from **Jeevan Asheesh Samiti** and the YouTube channel **Dietitian Ki Salah** have been instrumental in shaping this book into a comprehensive guide that caters to individuals from all walks of life. We are deeply grateful to both organizations for their unwavering commitment to promoting health, wellness, and mindful living.

We envision this book as a valuable resource for individuals seeking to embrace the transformative power of yoga and meditation. Designed to serve as a comprehensive guide, it is intended for students, academicians, health and wellness professionals, public health specialists, community development experts, program managers of national and international organizations, and practitioners at all levels. It is also an excellent addition to the libraries of relevant institutions and organizations promoting holistic well-being.

With heartfelt gratitude, we extend our sincere thanks to all the contributing authors for sharing their wisdom, experiences, and insights into the profound realms of yoga and meditation. Their efforts have greatly enriched the depth and practical value of this book. We believe this work is a significant step in addressing the growing need for mindfulness, inner peace, and well-being in today's fast-paced world.

As you embark on the journey through these pages, we hope that *Soulful Serenity* becomes a source of inspiration, guiding you toward a life of tranquility, emotional resilience, and profound inner peace. May **it inspire you to embrace yoga and meditation** not just as practices, but as lifelong companions on your path to well-being.

Happy reading! We look forward to receiving your insights and reflections.

Dr. Khushboo Gupta
Dr. Gopeswar Mukherjee
Dr. Sparsha Deep EM
Dr. Sangeeta
Dr. Vamshi Krishna Kondle

Publisher's Note

We are delighted to present ***Soulful Serenity: Yoga and Meditation for Blissful Life***, a transformative guide to living a life of peace, balance, and holistic well-being. In today's fast-paced and often stressful world, this book offers a sanctuary of wisdom and practical tools to help individuals reconnect with their inner selves, cultivate mindfulness, and foster long-lasting tranquility.

The authors have crafted a comprehensive and accessible resource that integrates the ancient teachings of yoga with modern-day needs. From enhancing physical health through asanas to calming the mind with meditation and pranayama, this book is a complete roadmap to achieving harmony in mind, body, and soul. Whether you are a novice or an experienced practitioner, the insights and practices shared within these pages will deepen your understanding of yoga and meditation, while offering you the opportunity to cultivate emotional resilience, mental clarity, and spiritual growth.

The approach taken in *Soulful Serenity* is both practical and profound, blending timeless wisdom with contemporary science, and offering guidance for readers at every stage of life. The focus on yoga's application in different life stages—from childhood to old age—and its benefits for pregnant women and new mothers makes this book a versatile and inclusive resource for all. Moreover, the sections dedicated to the science behind yoga's impact on stress and health will help readers experience the full potential of these transformative practices.

In addition, *Soulful Serenity* brings attention to the global celebration of yoga, including the significance of International Yoga Day, and emphasizes how yoga and meditation can create a peaceful and sustainable future for individuals and the world at large. The author's dedication to teaching holistic well-being shines through, making this book not just a guide, but a way of life.

We hope that *Soulful Serenity* inspires you to embark on your own journey of inner peace, mental clarity, and blissful living. May the teachings within these pages empower you to embrace yoga and meditation as essential practices that nourish your body, mind, and soul, and lead you to a more serene and joyful life.

We are proud to bring this valuable resource to our readers, and we trust that *Soulful Serenity* will be a cherished companion on your path to well-being.

With Regards

Hemakshee Publication

Biography
(Dr. Khushboo Gupta)

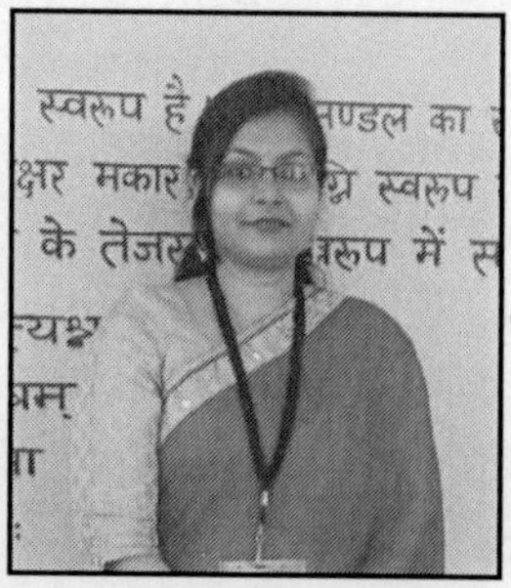

Dr. Khushboo Gupta is a PhD Home Science (Food Science and Nutrition) from Banasthali Vidyapith, Newai, India. She has been teaching subject including food chemistry, food analysis, therapeutic nutrition, human nutrition, human physiology and community nutrition, etc. Presently she is working as Assistant Professor in Trilok Singh TT College, Laxmangarh, Sikar, Rajasthan.

She is MSc Gold medalist and had **cleared UGC-NET and RPSC-SET examination.** Dr Gupta holds Advance Diploma in French Language from Banasthali Vidyapith; Diploma in Naturopathy and Yoga (NDDY) from Gandhi Smarak Prakritik Chikitsa Samiti (Regd.), New Delhi; Certificate in Homeopathic Medicinal System conducted by Vardhman Mahaveer Open University, Kota and Certificate in Statistical Techniques and Applications. She has featured in several programs of All India Radio and Radio Banasthali (FM 90.4).

Dr. Khushboo is actively involved in community activities especially those concerned with self-employment, health and wellness, optimum nutrition and how to improve quality of life of a person and family. She is the keynote speaker and founder of her YouTube channel "Dietitian Ki

Salah" through which she provides education related to optimum health, wellness and nutrition to masses. Dr. Gupta has published about more than 30 research papers in reputed national and international journals; 20 book chapters in different edited books, several news paper and magazine articles related to health, nutrition and new food product formulation. She authored two books related to elderly nutrition; edited **twenty two** books related to community science, food science and nutrition, health and wellness, issues with girls, health for all, sustainable development, food safety and security, breastfeeding, skill inculcation, Inflammatory bowel disease and millets for upliftment of the individuals of the society. She presented her research work in more than 26 national and international conferences. Her research is primarily in the area of food processing entrepreneurial skill Inculcation and geriatric nutrition. **The patent office, Government of India has granted a patent to Dr. Khushboo for her research on food formulation using RSM.** Dr. Gupta has successfully completed more than 30 courses on various diverse topics organized by SWAYAM, UNICEF, WHO and Cornell University.

In past she had worked as Assistant Professor (Food and Nutrition) in Modi University, Laxmangarh, Sikar; worked as Master Trainer in Agriculture University, Kota. During her PhD she had worked as UGC- SRF in Banasthali Vidyapith, Newai. One feather in her cap is that she had worked as regular trainee dietitian in dietetics department of Post Graduate Institute of Medical Education and Research (PGIMER), Chandigarh and got her short-term attachment certificate. She won many awards in different seminars and conferences for her contribution in scientific world. Apart from them, she is rewarded with **Teacher Honour award** by

Lions Club Kota South (September, 2017); '**Award of Honour**' given by All Rajasthan Qualified Homoeopathic Doctors Association in Homoeopathic Scientific Seminar, 2017, **Excellence Academician Award** given by Akhil Bhartiya Agrawal Mahasabha (Reg), Kota Branch (2023) and **Shakti Vandan Award** given by S.R.S.T. College of Education Ova Jahanabad, Bihar in association with Kalindi Prakashan, Ajamgarh, UP (2024).

She is the life member of many reputed institutes i.e. Nutrition Society of India, Indian Dietetic Association, The Indian Science Congress Association and Institute of Scholars and giving her services for upliftment of community.

Biography
(Dr. Gopeswar Mukharjee)

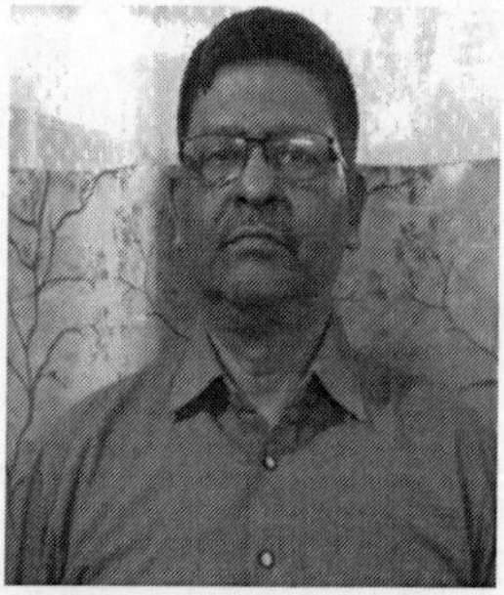

Gopeswar Mukharjee M.B.B.S., D.C.P., M.D. (Path.), Ph. D. (Path). Dsc (hon) is presently working as the Professor & dean of Brainware University, Kolkata.

He has an experience of working for more than 20 years as pathologist in WBHS & more than 12 yrs as M.O including MOIC in Blood Bank. He is trained on HLA Techniques from AIIMS, New Delhi & Molecular Genetics pathology from Kolkata, W.B and trained on Laboratory Diagnosis of Hemophilia conducted by Hemophilia Federation (India). Past working status of him are as follows: (i) Hony consultant pathologist of NH-Multi Speciality Hospital, Barasat; (ii) Hony consultant pathologist of Barasat Cancer Hospital; (iii) Ex-Pathologist and Guest Lecturer, Department of Pathology, Institute of Post Graduate Ay. Education & Research at SVSP, Kolkata, Govt. of West Bengal; (iv) Co-Supervisor of Ay. Post Graduate Students (M.D.) of the University of Calcutta and West Bengal University of health sciences, (v) Co-Supervisor of Ph. D. programme.

He wrote books and multiple papers in national and international scientific journals and presented his work in various conferences and seminars

Biography
(Dr Sparsha Deep EM)

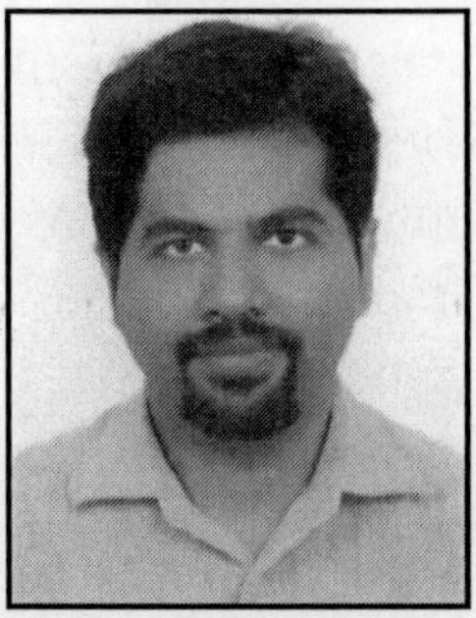

Dr Sparsha Deep EM is currently the Professor & Head, Department of Pharmacology and Chief Coordinator of Clinical Skills & Simulation Lab at Shridevi Institute of Medical Sciences & Research Hospital (SIMS&RH), Tumakuru, Karnataka. He has been serving in the field of medical education, research & clinical practice for the last 15 years. He is a certified Emergency Care & Life Support (ECLS) trainer from Jeeva Raksha Trust, Bengaluru. He has previously given his services in reputed institutions like A J Institute of Medical Sciences & Research Centre (AJIMS&RC), Mangalore, and Govt. Medical College (GMC) Kannur, Kerala.

He has been awarded M-FILIPE (FAIMER) Fellowship from MAHE, Manipal (2021); Advanced Course in Medical Education (ACME) form GMC, Kottayam, Kerala (2016). Dr Sparsha Deep EM has to his credits publications in indexed peer reviewed journals. His areas of expertise are Pharmacotherapeutics; Pharmacovigilance; Clinical Research & ICH- GCP (Good Clinical Practice) and Medical Humanities. He has received Jury Choice award for his presentation on topic 'Clinical simulation in the learning of management of anaphylaxis in medical undergraduates' at JIPMER MEDUCON 2021.

Biography

(Dr. Sangeeta)

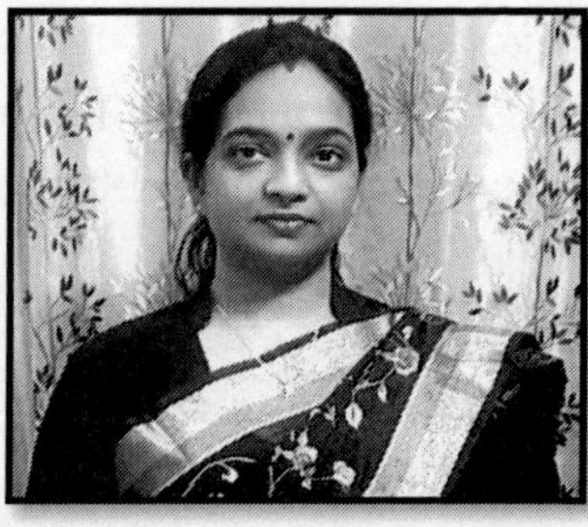

Dr. Sangeeta is working as Assistant Professor in Home-Science (Food & Nutrition) at Ramabai Govt. Women Post Graduate College- Akbarpur, Ambedkar nagar- Uttar-Pradesh. She has 13 year experience of teaching to graduates and Post graduate students. She Qualifies the U. G. C. NET Examination in June 2005. Her more than 35 research papers have been published in National and International Journals and Proceedings of seminars as well as 12 Book chapters published from National and International Publishers. She has more than 10 societies and institutional life Membership

She got many prestigious awards such as Best Teacher Award, Young Scientist Award; Award from Higher Education, Excellence Academician Award, Best Oral Presentation Award etc. she had organized 6 webinars and 07 International Conferences. She was the member of organizing committees of 2 national conferences. She wrote 2 books and edited 6 books. She is the member and coordinator of various college committees including IQAC. Dr. Sangeeta presented her papers in about 23 International conferences and 25 national conferences.

Biography

(Dr Vamshi krishna Kondle)

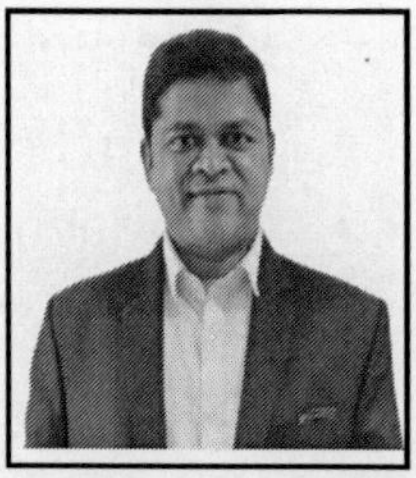

Renowned academician, teacher, researcher, author ,and editor with 20 years' experience in the field of Child Health Care, Medical education, Research, and Publication. Presently working as Vice Dean and Professor & HOD of Pediatrics at RVM Institute of medical sciences and Research centre, India. Dr Vamshi Kondle received national and international recognition in the fields of Child Health, Medical Education, and clinical research. Served as technical expert/advisor on policy making and research to Government of Telangana Published 12 papers National /international journals in indexed journals. Editorial committee Member of Indian Academy of Pediatrics twin cities branch for 2 years 2021-22. Member of IAP, IMA, AME, and IAPNRC, IAP ID , ICANCL ,

Received National and international awards and recognition for child health and Research, trained thousands of MBBS and hundreds of postgraduates. He was selected as the Academic Senate member at KNRUHS. Actively involved in research and training of health professionals and community for rational management Of child diseases and essential newborn health through IAP being an official Spokesperson of "IAP ke baat community ke saath". Served different positions as Executive member, state and TCB Treasurer, twin cities branch, Secretary General & state Vice-President State ,In IAP .President IMA, kompally .

List of Contributors

- **Dr. Khushboo Gupta**, Assistant Professor, Trilok Singh TT College, Lakshmangarh, Sikar (Rajasthan), India
- **Dr. Suresh Kumar Agarwal**, M.Sc. (Yoga), M.D. (Homoeo), Ph.D., Director, International Institute of Lifestyle Medicine
- **Surbhee Gupta**, Assistant at LIC of India
- **Dr. S. Abdul Jabbar**, Assistant Professor, Dept. of Education and Training, MANUU, Hyderabad
- **Dr Shraddha Thacker**, Assistant Professor, Dept. of Human Development, L.A.D. and Smt. R.P College for Women, Nagpur
- **Mrs. Arti Negi**, Assistant professor, SGRRIM&HS, COLLEGE OF NURSING
- **Rohini Chourasiya**, Govt. Girls College, Vidisha
- **CA Dinesh Agrawal**, FCA, B.Com, Sikar, Rajasthan
- **Dr. Lok Mani Gupta**, Homoeopathic Doctor, Gupta Homoeo Clinic, Kota Rajasthan
- **Saurabh Gupta**, Assistant Manager, UCO Bank, Bijainagar
- **Minkal Tuteja**, Panipat Institute of Engineering and Technology, Samalkha Panipat, Haryana-132102

- **Anil Kuntal,** Assistant professor, FIITJEE Ltd., Delhi
- **Shivani Khare** (Home Science), Government Girls Post Graduate College, Satna (M.P.)
- **Jyoti Dahiya,** Self-Financing Guest Scholar (Home Science Department), Government Girls Post Graduate College, Satna (M.P.)
- **Dr. Amrita Singh,** Assistant Professor, Department of Home Science, IGNTU Amarkantak

If readers have any query related to any chapter of the book, kindly contact with the corresponding author of the chapter. Authors of the chapters are solely responsible for their work.

1.

International Yoga Day - History & Importance

Dr. Suresh Kumar Agarwal,

M.Sc. (Yoga), M.D. (Homoeo), Ph.D.

Director, International Institute of Lifestyle Medicine

Email: drskagarwal3333@gmail.com

1. History of International Yoga Day

International Yoga Day is celebrated annually on June 21st. The idea of an international day to celebrate yoga was first proposed by India and has grown into a global observance. Here is a brief history of how it came into being:

September 27, 2014: Indian Prime Minister Narendra Modi proposed the idea of an International Day of Yoga during his speech at the United Nations General Assembly (UNGA). In his address, he highlighted yoga's universal appeal, describing it as an invaluable gift from India's ancient tradition. Narendra Modi emphasized that yoga embodies unity of mind and body, thought and action, restraint and fulfillment, and harmony between humans and nature. He suggested that an international day dedicated to yoga would help promote healthier lifestyles and global well-being.

December 11, 2014: Following Narendra Modi's proposal, the UNGA adopted Resolution 69/131, which proclaimed June 21st as the International Day of Yoga. The resolution was endorsed by a record 177 member states, reflecting the widespread support and recognition of yoga's benefits. The date of June 21st was chosen because it is the summer solstice, the longest day of the year in the Northern Hemisphere, which holds special significance in many parts of the world and symbolizes light, life, and the potential for new beginnings.

June 21, 2015: The first International Day of Yoga was celebrated globally with great enthusiasm. In India, the main event took place in New Delhi, where Prime Minister Narendra Modi led a mass yoga demonstration attended by thousands of people, including government officials, diplomats, and citizens from various walks of life. This event set two Guinness World Records: one for the largest yoga class, with 35,985 participants, and another for the most nationalities participating in a single yoga session, with people from 84 different countries. Globally, numerous events were organized to mark the occasion. Yoga sessions were held in various countries, from large public parks to community centers, schools, and private homes, demonstrating the universal appeal of yoga.

2. Importance of International Yoga Day and Why We Need It

International Yoga Day holds significant importance for several reasons, reflecting the multifaceted benefits of yoga for individuals and societies globally. During his speech at the United Nations General Assembly (UNGA) on September 27, 2014, Indian Prime Minister Narendra Modi emphasized the importance and benefits of yoga. Here are some key quotes from his proposal:

- On Yoga's Universal Appeal - "Yoga is an invaluable gift of India's ancient tradition. This tradition is 5,000 years old. It embodies unity of mind and body; thought and action; restraint and fulfillment; harmony between man and nature; a holistic approach to health and well-being."
- On Promoting Well-being - "Yoga is not just about exercise; it is a way to discover the sense of oneness with yourself, the world, and nature."
- On Choosing an International Day - "By changing our lifestyle and creating consciousness, it can help us deal with climate change. Let us work towards adopting an International Yoga Day."

These statements highlight Modi's belief in yoga's potential to foster global well-being, harmony, and environmental consciousness, advocating for its worldwide recognition and practice.

3. Why We Need Such A Day?

Yoga is a holistic practice that integrates physical postures, breathing techniques, and meditation to promote overall health and well-being. Regular practice of yoga can lead to improved physical fitness and flexibility, enhanced mental clarity and emotional balance, reduced stress and anxiety, better cardiovascular and respiratory health, enhanced immune function. By dedicating a day to yoga, people are encouraged to incorporate these beneficial practices into their daily lives, leading to healthier lifestyles and a reduction in lifestyle-related diseases.

In the modern world, mental health issues such as stress, anxiety, and depression are on the rise. Yoga offers tools to manage and alleviate these conditions. International Yoga Day brings attention to the mental health benefits of yoga, encouraging individuals to use these practices to improve their mental well-being. Yoga is an inclusive practice that can be adapted to suit people of all ages, abilities, and fitness levels. By promoting yoga through an international observance, we highlight its accessibility and adaptability, encouraging more people to participate and benefit from its practices. Promoting yoga on a global scale can have economic benefits as well. It can boost tourism in regions known for yoga retreats and training centers. Additionally, the wellness industry, including yoga studios, apparel, and accessories, can experience growth as more people take up the practice.

International Yoga Day serves as a reminder of the numerous benefits of yoga and encourages individuals to incorporate these practices into their daily lives. It promotes health, well-being, and unity, while also preserving an ancient cultural heritage and fostering environmental consciousness. By celebrating this day, we acknowledge the importance of a holistic approach to health and promote a more balanced and harmonious way of living.

4. Why is International Yoga Day celebrated on June 21st?

International Yoga Day is celebrated on June 21st because it is the day of the summer solstice, which holds special significance in many parts of the world. Here are the key reasons why this date was chosen:

- **Longest Day of the Year**: June 21st is the longest day of the year in the Northern Hemisphere. It marks the summer solstice, a time when the tilt of Earth's axis is most inclined towards the sun, resulting in the maximum hours of daylight.

- **Symbolism of Light**: The summer solstice is often associated with light and enlightenment, symbolizing the triumph of light over darkness. This symbolism aligns with the essence of yoga, which aims to bring clarity, balance, and harmony to one's life.

- **Ancient Practices**: Many ancient civilizations, including those in India, have celebrated the summer solstice as a time of spiritual significance. In Indian tradition, it is believed that the first transmission of yoga by Lord Shiva to his disciples began on this day.

- **Support and Consensus**: The choice of June 21st received widespread support from UN member states. The endorsement by 177 member countries in the resolution highlights the consensus on the significance of this date for celebrating yoga.

When proposing International Yoga Day at the United Nations General Assembly on September 27, 2014,

Prime Minister Narendra Modi highlighted the importance of the summer solstice in choosing the date : "The date of the summer solstice is the longest day of the year in the Northern Hemisphere and has special significance in many parts of the world. It is considered as a time when nature is in its fullest expression, and it represents the transition to Dakshinayana, which is significant in the yogic tradition."

By aligning International Yoga Day with the summer solstice, the day celebrates not only the physical and mental benefits of yoga but also its deep philosophical and spiritual roots that connect humans with the natural world.

5. Themes of International Yoga Day

- 2015 : Yoga for Harmony and Peace
- 2016 : Connect the Youth
- 2017 : Yoga for Health
- 2018 : Yoga for Peace
- 2019 : Yoga for Heart
- 2020 : Yoga at Home and Yoga with Family
- 2021 : Yoga for Well-being
- 2022 : Yoga for Humanity
- 2023 : Yoga for Vasudhaiva Kutumbakam
- 2024 : Yoga for Self and Society

6. Role of Swami Amrita Suryananda Saraswati in International Yoga Day

Swami Amrita Suryananda Saraswati, also known as Amritaji, is a renowned spiritual leader and yoga teacher who has made significant contributions to the promotion and practice of yoga worldwide. His spiritual journey began early in life, driven by a deep-seated quest for knowledge and spiritual realization. He studied under various spiritual masters and received extensive training in yoga, Vedanta, and meditation. His profound understanding of these ancient teachings forms the basis of his teachings and practices today. He is associated with Portugal. He has been actively involved in spreading the teachings of yoga and spirituality in Portugal and beyond. Swami Amrita Suryananda Saraswati has established yoga centers, conducted workshops, and led spiritual retreats in Portugal, contributing significantly to the growth of yoga community and awareness in the country. His teachings emphasize a holistic approach to yoga, encompassing physical, mental, and spiritual aspects, and have garnered a following among practitioners seeking deeper spiritual understanding and personal growth.

Amritaji has played an active role in promoting International Yoga Day and its objectives. He has been instrumental in organizing large-scale yoga events, workshops, and seminars both in India and internationally. These events aim to raise awareness about the benefits of yoga and encourage people from all walks of life to adopt yoga as a way of life. Amritaji's presence at these gatherings inspires participants to deepen their practice and integrate yoga into their daily routines. As a teacher, he emphasizes the holistic approach of yoga, which encompasses physical postures (asanas), breathing techniques (pranayama), meditation, and ethical principles (yamas and niyamas). His teachings focus not only on physical health but also on mental clarity, emotional balance, and spiritual awakening. He encourages his students to explore yoga as a tool for self-discovery and inner transformation, guiding them on a journey towards self-realization and spiritual enlightenment.

Swami Amrita Suryananda Saraswati's role in promoting yoga, especially in the context of International Yoga Day, underscores his commitment to sharing the timeless wisdom of yoga for personal and collective transformation. His teachings embody the essence of yoga as a path to inner peace, harmony, and spiritual fulfillment.

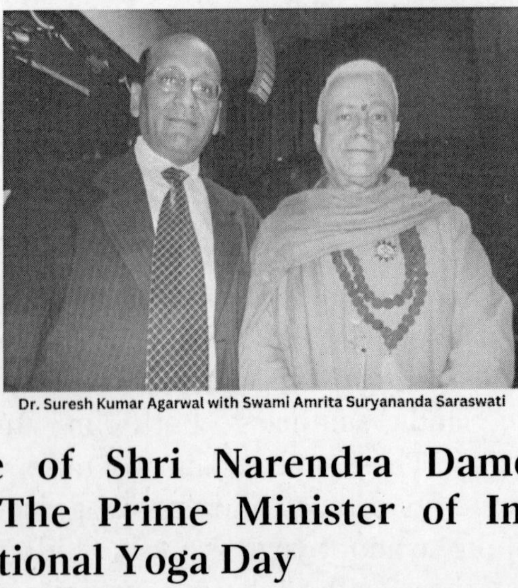

Dr. Suresh Kumar Agarwal with Swami Amrita Suryananda Saraswati

7. Role of Shri Narendra Damodardas Modi (The Prime Minister of India) in International Yoga Day

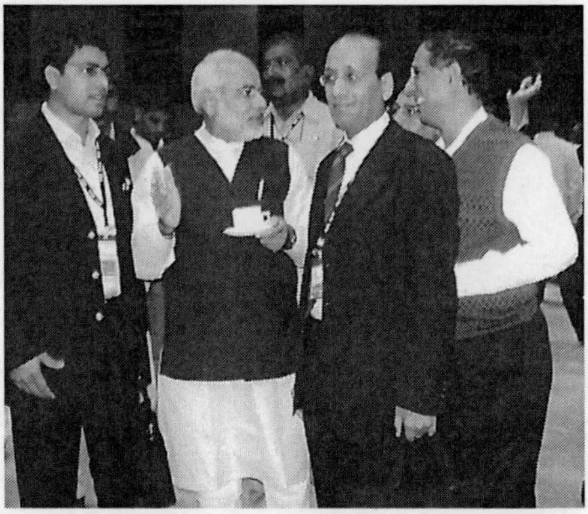

Shri Narendra Damodardas Modi, the Prime Minister of India, has played a pivotal role in the establishment and global recognition of International Yoga Day. His leadership and advocacy have significantly contributed to the promotion of yoga as a universal practice for health, harmony, and spiritual well-being.

Prime Minister Narendra Modi proposed the idea of International Yoga Day during his address to the United Nations General Assembly (UNGA) on September 27, 2014. In his speech, Modi highlighted yoga's ancient roots in Indian culture and its universal appeal as a holistic practice that integrates physical, mental, and spiritual dimensions. He emphasized yoga's potential to promote individual well-being and global harmony, presenting it as a means to achieve a healthier and more peaceful world. Following his proposal, the UNGA adopted Resolution 69/131 on December 11, 2014, proclaiming June 21st as International Day of Yoga. This resolution received unprecedented support from 177 member states, underscoring the global consensus on the significance of yoga and its benefits. Narendra Modi's diplomatic efforts and persuasive advocacy were instrumental in garnering international support for the resolution, making International Yoga Day a globally recognized observance.

Since its inception, Narendra Modi has actively participated in and led the celebrations of International Yoga Day in India. The inaugural International Yoga Day on June 21, 2015, witnessed a historic event in New Delhi, where Modi himself led a mass yoga session attended by thousands of people, including government officials, diplomats, and citizens. This event not only set Guinness World Records for the largest yoga class and the most nationalities participating in a yoga session but also symbolized his personal commitment to promoting yoga as a national and global heritage. Under Narendra Modi's leadership, the Indian government has continued to promote yoga through various initiatives and programs. These efforts include organizing yoga workshops, seminars, and demonstrations across India and abroad, aimed at raising awareness about yoga's physical, mental, and spiritual benefits.

In essence, Narendra Modi's vision and leadership have been instrumental in elevating yoga to a global platform through International Yoga Day. His advocacy has not only popularized yoga as a lifestyle choice but also underscored its potential to contribute to individual well-being, global health, and international cooperation.

2.

The Essence of Yoga: Union of Body, Mind, and Soul

Surbhee Gupta

Assistant at LIC of India

Email: sb7529@gmail.com

Yoga, derived from the Sanskrit word "Yuj," meaning union or to join, is an ancient practice rooted in Indian philosophy. It is both a science and an art of living, aimed at achieving harmony among the body, mind, and soul.

1. The Philosophy of Yoga

At its core, yoga is a path to self-realization and inner peace. Originating over 5,000 years ago, yoga integrates physical postures (asanas), breath control (pranayama), and meditation (dhyana) to transcend the limitations of the mind and body. Central to its philosophy are the following key principles:

1. **Unity in Diversity:** Yoga teaches the interconnectedness of all living beings and emphasizes the union of the individual self (Atman) with the universal consciousness (Brahman).

2. **The Eightfold Path of Patanjali:** Outlined in the Yoga Sutras, Patanjali's Ashtanga Yoga provides a

comprehensive framework for spiritual growth and self-realization. The eight limbs are:

- **Yama (Ethical Principles):** These are moral restraints or guidelines for interactions with others and the world, promoting virtues like non-violence (Ahimsa), truthfulness (Satya), non-stealing (Asteya), chastity (Brahmacharya), and non-possessiveness (Aparigraha).
- **Niyama (Personal Discipline):** These are observances for personal growth and inner discipline, including cleanliness (Shaucha), contentment (Santosha), self-discipline (Tapas), self-study (Swadhyaya), and surrender to a higher power (Ishwar-Pranidhana).
- **Asana (Postures):** Physical postures prepare the body for prolonged meditation by promoting strength, flexibility, and comfort. The practice of asanas also ensures physical well-being.
- **Pranayama (Breath Control):** Techniques for controlling the breath regulate the flow of vital energy (prana) in the body, enhancing mental clarity and emotional stability.
- **Pratyahara (Withdrawal of Senses):** This practice involves turning inward by detaching the senses from external distractions, fostering a heightened sense of awareness and focus.
- **Dharana (Concentration):** Concentrating the mind on a single object or thought, such as a mantra or a flame, helps develop mental discipline and reduce distractions.

- **Dhyana (Meditation):** Meditation deepens the focus achieved in Dharana, leading to a continuous flow of contemplation and inner peace.
- **Samadhi (Blissful Union):** The ultimate goal of yoga, Samadhi is a state of spiritual enlightenment and union with the universal consciousness, transcending the ego and worldly concerns.

3. **Holistic Well-being:** Yoga is not limited to physical fitness but extends to emotional and spiritual growth, fostering a balanced life.

2. The Concept of Holistic Wellness

Holistic wellness refers to a state of complete physical, mental, emotional, social, and spiritual well-being. Unlike conventional approaches that often focus on treating specific ailments, holistic wellness emphasizes prevention, balance, and integration across all aspects of life. It acknowledges that the body, mind, and spirit are deeply interconnected and that harmony among these elements is essential for optimal health.

Holistic wellness encompasses the following dimensions:

1. **Physical Wellness:** Maintaining a healthy body through proper nutrition, regular exercise, adequate sleep, and preventive care.
2. **Mental Wellness:** Developing cognitive resilience, managing stress effectively, and cultivating a positive mindset.

3. **Emotional Wellness:** Acknowledging, processing, and expressing emotions in a healthy manner, fostering emotional intelligence and balance.
4. **Social Wellness:** Building meaningful relationships and maintaining a supportive social network.
5. **Spiritual Wellness:** Connecting with one's inner self and the larger universe, exploring purpose, and embracing values that provide meaning to life.

3. Achieving Holistic Wellness Through Yoga

Yoga serves as a powerful tool for achieving holistic wellness by addressing all dimensions of well-being:

1. **Physical Wellness Through Asanas:**
   - Regular practice of asanas improves strength, flexibility, and posture.
   - It enhances physiological functions such as digestion, circulation, and immune response.
   - Examples include Tadasana (Mountain Pose) for alignment, Vrikshasana (Tree Pose) for balance, and Bhujangasana (Cobra Pose) for spinal health.
2. **Mental Wellness Through Pranayama:**
   - Breath control practices regulate the autonomic nervous system, reducing stress and promoting relaxation.
   - Techniques like Nadi Shodhana (alternate nostril breathing) and Bhramari (humming bee breath) calm the mind and improve focus.

3. **Emotional Wellness Through Meditation:**
    - Meditation fosters self-awareness, emotional regulation, and a sense of inner peace.
    - Guided meditations, mindfulness practices, and yoga nidra help individuals process emotions and cultivate gratitude and compassion.
4. **Social Wellness Through Karma Yoga:**
    - The path of selfless service encourages acts of kindness and empathy, strengthening community bonds.
    - Group yoga classes and retreats provide opportunities for social interaction and collective growth.
5. **Spiritual Wellness Through Dhyana and Bhakti Yoga:**
    - Meditation (Dhyana) deepens one's connection with the higher self.
    - Bhakti Yoga, the path of devotion, nurtures spiritual growth through prayer, chanting, and rituals.

4. Practical Steps to Integrate Yoga for Holistic Wellness

1. **Daily Routine:** Begin with 15-20 minutes of gentle stretches and breathing exercises, gradually increasing the duration and intensity.

2. **Mindful Eating:** Adopt a sattvic diet rich in fresh, wholesome, and plant-based foods that nourish the body and mind.

3. **Stress Management:** Incorporate short meditation sessions or pranayama techniques during breaks to reset and recharge.

4. **Community Engagement:** Participate in group yoga sessions, workshops, or volunteer activities to foster social connections.

5. **Personal Reflection:** Maintain a journal to record insights, intentions, and areas of growth.

6. **Seek Guidance:** Work with a qualified yoga instructor or mentor to develop a personalized practice tailored to individual needs.

5. The Physical Aspect: Body

Yoga asanas are designed to maintain the physical body—the vehicle through which individuals experience the world. Key benefits include:

1. **Improved Flexibility and Strength:** Regular practice enhances muscle tone, joint mobility, and overall stamina.

2. **Health and Wellness:** Yoga supports cardiovascular health, boosts immunity, and aids in the management of chronic conditions such as diabetes and arthritis.

3. **Detoxification:** Twisting, bending, and stretching postures help stimulate the body's internal organs and promote detoxification.

Popular asanas like Tadasana (Mountain Pose), Trikonasana (Triangle Pose), and Savasana (Corpse Pose) demonstrate the diversity of yoga postures aimed at aligning the body's energy. Additionally, poses like Bhujangasana (Cobra Pose) and Adho Mukha Svanasana (Downward Dog Pose) offer targeted benefits for specific muscle groups.

6. The Mental Aspect: Mind

Yoga addresses mental health through techniques that calm the mind and improve focus. The mental benefits of yoga include:

1. **Stress Reduction:** Practices such as pranayama and meditation activate the parasympathetic nervous system, reducing cortisol levels and alleviating anxiety.
2. **Enhanced Concentration and Memory:** Yoga helps sharpen mental clarity and focus, benefiting both academic and professional pursuits.
3. **Emotional Balance:** Through mindfulness, yoga encourages acceptance, self-awareness, and resilience. It aids in managing emotions and cultivating a positive outlook.

Techniques such as Nadi Shodhana (alternate nostril breathing), Kapalabhati (cleansing breath), and mindful meditation are powerful tools for cultivating a tranquil mind. Regular practice of Trataka (focused gazing) also strengthens concentration and mental discipline.

7. The Spiritual Aspect: Soul

Yoga's ultimate goal is spiritual liberation—the realization of one's true nature beyond physical and mental limitations. Spiritual benefits include:

1. **Inner Peace:** By silencing the fluctuations of the mind, yoga enables individuals to experience profound stillness and a connection to their inner self.
2. **Self-Realization:** Regular practice fosters a connection with the higher self and the universe, leading to a sense of purpose and meaning.
3. **Compassion and Oneness:** Yoga practitioners often develop a heightened sense of empathy and interconnectedness with all living beings.

Bhakti Yoga (path of devotion), Jnana Yoga (path of knowledge), and Karma Yoga (path of selfless action) illustrate how yoga transcends physical practices to nurture the soul. These paths provide unique approaches for individuals to achieve spiritual growth based on their temperament and life circumstances.

8. Integration: Body, Mind, and Soul

Yoga is most impactful when it fosters a seamless connection between the physical, mental, and spiritual realms. Achieving this integration requires an intentional practice that harmonizes movement, breath, and awareness. Here's how yoga unites these three dimensions:

1. **Synergy Through Asana and Pranayama:**
   - Physical postures (asanas) prepare the body by strengthening it and making it more flexible,

while breath control (pranayama) enhances energy flow, linking the physical form with the mind's rhythm.

  - Practices like Sun Salutations (Surya Namaskar) are dynamic sequences that synchronize breath and movement, creating a meditative flow.

2. **Mindful Meditation:**
   - Meditation bridges the mind and soul, calming mental chatter and allowing practitioners to access deeper states of consciousness.
   - Techniques like mindfulness and transcendental meditation create a space for introspection, aligning thoughts with higher aspirations.

3. **Spiritual Awakening:**
   - By transcending physical and mental limitations, yoga encourages practitioners to connect with their true self.
   - Chanting mantras such as "Om" or performing devotional practices enhance this connection, fostering a sense of oneness with the universe.

4. **Balancing the Chakras:**
   - Yoga also integrates the subtle energy system by balancing the chakras (energy centers). For instance, grounding poses like Warrior II stabilize the root chakra (Muladhara), while heart-opening poses like Camel (Ustrasana) activate the heart chakra (Anahata).

5. **Holistic Practices:**

- Practices such as Yoga Nidra (yogic sleep) combine physical relaxation, mental clarity, and spiritual awareness, offering a complete experience of integration.

9. Practical Applications

Yoga is not merely a theoretical discipline but a practical way of living. Its benefits extend to every aspect of daily life, promoting physical vitality, mental clarity, and spiritual balance. Here are some suggestions for incorporating yoga into your daily routine:

1. **Morning Routine:**
   - Begin the day with gentle stretches to awaken the body, such as Cat-Cow Pose (Marjaryasana-Bitilasana) and Child's Pose (Balasana).
   - Practice mindful breathing, like Nadi Shodhana (alternate nostril breathing), to calm the mind and set a positive tone for the day.
   - Include a short sequence of Sun Salutations (Surya Namaskar) to energize the body and mind.
2. **Midday Breaks:**
   - Take 5–10 minutes to practice chair yoga or simple stretches at your desk to relieve tension in the shoulders, back, and neck.
   - Perform quick pranayama techniques, such as Bhramari (humming bee breath), to restore focus and reduce midday stress.

- Incorporate mindfulness by stepping outside for a brief walking meditation or grounding exercise.

3. **Evening Relaxation:**
    - Wind down with restorative yoga poses, such as Legs-Up-The-Wall Pose (Viparita Karani) or Reclining Butterfly Pose (Supta Baddha Konasana).
    - Practice a guided meditation or Yoga Nidra to release stress and promote deep relaxation.
    - End the day with a gratitude practice, reflecting on positive moments and setting intentions for restful sleep.

By integrating these practices into everyday life, yoga becomes a seamless part of your routine, fostering a balanced and harmonious lifestyle.

10. Conclusions

The essence of yoga lies in its ability to unite body, mind, and soul, leading to a state of holistic well-being and self-realization. By incorporating physical postures, mindful breathing, and meditative awareness, yoga becomes a powerful tool for transformation. Its teachings transcend physical exercise, offering a pathway to inner peace, harmony, and spiritual awakening. In embracing yoga as a lifestyle, individuals can achieve a profound balance, experiencing life with heightened awareness and connection to the self and the universe.

3

Integral Yoga Education

Dr. S. Abdul Jabbar

Assistant Professor

Dept. of Education and Training, MANUU, Hyderabad

Email: jabbaragatti@gmail.com,

Abstract

For embedding education with mindfulness, social justice teaching, and holistic development, this article explores the scope for new yoga-integrated pedagogy. Neither does the old typical class allow students to elevate a discussion on critical issues nor adjudicate their non-scholastic outcomes. Nevertheless, this new approach gives freedom to students to explore their experiences collaboratively and rule out overwhelming mental trauma and other negative connotations. It will enable action-oriented, open-minded, unorthodox, and cosmopolitan narratives. In this article, we explore thenew concept of yoga integration in the classroom teaching and learning process and its benefits. It also includes some tips for teachers to practice yoga-integrated pedagogy.

Keywords: Yoga-oriented Pedagogy, the significance of yoga integration and Yoga teaching tips.

1. Introduction

Yoga for the teaching and learning process has been triggering massive inputs recently. Probably a pleasant environment and a pretty fair direct instance of experiential learning and encountering a bunches of the stress-free environment in the class perhaps greater than typical bookish could be turn out or pops up the weird as well as giant crazy happiness relaxation is the main pertinence confronting while Integrating yoga pedagogy. Nevertheless, it underscores a couple of boosts for teachers and students in an astounding zeal that they will triumph in co-curricular or non-scholastic-related deeds. For teachers, it acquaints them with a comprehensive sense of prototype that enhances them to be more effective and skilled instructors.

2. Yoga-oriented Pedagogy

It is a breakthrough in pedagogy and practice to create an engaging and transformative class for their students, who seemed overshadowed and frustrated. The Comprehension of yoga integration into a typical classroom can be bloomed and overwhelmed with iconic experiences. What is required for social and personal life is perfectly articulated by a teacher about that knowledge. The perplexed child of mugging up the content can sign off their bewilderment and chaos and eventually can have an idea or archetype on the content which they are supposed to study. Acknowledging as well as endorsing

3. Significance of yoga integration

To develop ideal teacher skills for the 21st Century Continuous education in yoga is mandatory. Developing essential yoga pedagogy for teachers there should never be an environment of panic and turn out in a pretty awesome legacy. Training can be perfectly provided making them attend workshops, trainings, and conferences. It, of course, triggers or deepens their understanding and knowledge of fabulous yoga instructions. The other way of ensuring the training is in such a way that they can seek mentorship from experienced teachers and can acknowledge a kind of feedback that is incorporated into their teaching. Eventually, it enhances them to be an outstanding expert and the skills so far can debut in their new classroom. This of course can have a moment where you will feel scintillated about your performance and indeed will have a remarkable retention of happiness, enlightenment, optimization, and a spectrum of spectacular involvement with students and other colleagues.

Integration Yoga unfolds a new environment in the typical class, which has been scary for both teachers and the students so far. Perhaps there might be teachers who do not know how physical and mental health is important for learning. He or she indeed never thought of making students relax. Right not through the pretty good integration, learning probably elevates and the students can perceive the content without any embarrassment. Yoga helps pupils to have the following benefits:

- Yoga develops a student's completely integrated personality.
- It nurtures our life with proper values, and social and interpersonal skills not only in our classroom life but also outside the class.
- It is a key to treasure for an individual and the social life at large.
- It is equipped with the philosophy of practical life and emphasizes curative and therapeutic valuesthat can be extended to children in the school.
- This helps self-discipline in our individual lives and a balance in the workplace.
- It unfolds your inner peace and development of behaviors
- It creates relaxation mentally, physically, etc.

It plays a crucial role in the growth and development of students. It accelerates the teacher's incorporation of the key principles of content that they usually teach. This concept of new pedagogy ameliorates a great creative and supportive class. It nurtures students' feelings of health consciousness. It enhances an environment for exploring old ideas in a new platform. Students can feel and amplify their confidence and practice their course without stress and chaos.

4. Yoga Teaching Tips

The teacher should know that stress is everywhere in pupils' lives and influences their well-being at home and school. This new approach to yoga integration ought to reduce stress and mental chaos. However, at the same time usually in the school teachers typically have little time to add extra activities more than academics.Yoga can never only be a physically oriented practice, but it involves life-required skills and abilities. It is the pedagogical perspective that can connect a teacher with his or her students in a more sensible way, who leads their lives. To integrate yoga successfully into one's class, teachers should follow these suggested teaching tips.

- Keep yourself balanced always; physically and psychologically.
- Incorporate the art of breathing and other poses
- Commit yourself to practical classes or practices
- Keep learning new ideas
- Orient the students in a healthy way
- Help in adding students self-care and flexibility
- Involve in nurturing the skills of resilience and self-esteem
- Concentrate on pupils' attention span and deliberations
- Always think about the mental and physical health of students

Yoga education is embedded in a massive concept of becoming or creating a complete human being. There are interdisciplinary ideas by default rooted in yoga integration that we can encounter in the art and science of yoga. No option in and around yoga escalates a kind of spiritual realization and inner and social harmony.

The amazing concepts that are being manifested can enable students to shape their lives and build interpersonal relationships not only at school but also with the community. The primary thing we should adopt when a teacher trains and the concept of yoga and its practical classes can be included so that the school curriculum can easily deliver these interrogative pedagogical views. As far as the teacher and the student are concerned there is equal benefit not only psychologically but also holistically. The offshoot of this is seen in our emotional, social, and physical health.

5. Conclusions

Acquainting students with an explicitly integrated personality and their holistic development is a pertinent accomplishment of education. Either primary secondary, or higher education, it can be strengthened through the integration of yoga into our curriculum. Of course, it has been quite clear that a child in this modern technologically advanced world never has a chance to develop their social values, healthy hygienic life, and cognitive and mentally adjusted life. Nevertheless, to get rid of a child from this chaotic and crazy life of the modern, teachers can sign off this by understanding the integration of yoga into our syllabus and at large in the curriculum. Here it is required need right now to practice yoga in our school curriculum and higher studies as well. It is a mandatory fact that our teachers as well as classrooms ought to be equipped with the facilities.

References

1. A 21st-Century Yogasanalia: Celebrating the Integration of Yoga, Science, and Medicine. (2017). (n.p.): Wheatmark, Inc...

2. Cuomo, N. C. (2007). Integrated Yoga: Yoga with a Sensory Integrative Approach. United Kingdom: Jessica Kingsley Publishers.

3. Davies, A. (2016). Understanding modern Yoga pedagogy and curriculum: exploring sense-making by senior Western Yoga teacher-trainers (Doctoral dissertation, University of Southern Queensland).

4. Dr.S.Abdul Jabbar (2020) Sociological Concepts, Lambert Academic Publishing, Mauritius

5. Dr.S. Abdul Jabbar (2021) Guidance and counseling, Lambert Academic Publishing, Mauritius

4.

"प्राणस्यविज्ञानंजीवनस्यविज्ञानम्"- Understanding of Pran and Pranayam

Dr Shraddha Thacker

Assistant Professor,

Dept. of Human Development, L.A.D. and Smt. R.P College for Women, Nagpur

Email: shraddha_patelia@rediffmail.com

1. Introduction

We know that from womb to tomb our breathing process continues unabated. Breath and Praná are two different things altogether. But we cannot see them apart from each - other. Breath is Sthula (gross) and Praná is Suksham (Subtle). Breath is the external manifestation of Praná. Praná permeates everything and everywhere. It is through the agency of breath that we partake of this vital force ceaselessly. All the things of the world that have life, energy and mobility and mobility are infused with Praná. Man in Sanskrit is called Prani because he possesses Praná (Sharma and Suman, 1999, p. 123)

Pranáis a fundamental concept in ancient Indian philosophy, particularly within the disciplines of Yoga and Ayurveda and is believed to flow through channels called "Nadis" and is the foundation of all life and consciousness.It is the energy that powers our physical body, thoughts, emotions, and spiritual well-being. According to yogic traditions, there are five types of Prana known as "Pancha Pranas," each governing different functions of the body and mind:

1. **Prana:** This is the primary life force, associated with inhalation and energy intake. It governs the **respiratory system** and is primarily situated in the heart and lungs.

2. **Apana:** Associated with exhalation and the downward-moving energy, Apana governs **elimination processes**, including defecation, urination, and childbirth. It is located in the lower abdomen.

3. **Samana:** This type of Prana is linked with **digestion and assimilation** of food and nutrients. It is the balancing force that integrates and regulates energy. Samana is situated in the region of the navel.

4. **Udana:** Udana is responsible for **sound production**, speech, and growth. It governs the functions of the throat and neck and helps maintain our energy levels. It is associated with the upward-moving energy.

5. **Vyana:** This type of Prana circulates throughout the body, managing the overall coordination and movement. It governs **circulation,** the nervous system, and the distribution of energy to every cell.

Understanding the roles of different types of Prana is crucial for achieving physical, mental, and spiritual harmony. Imbalances or blockages in the flow of Prana can lead to illness, stress, and other health issues. This is where the practice of Pranayam comes into play.

The word pranayama is formed by two words i.e., prana and ayama. 'Prana' means a subtle life force, which provides energy to different organs (including mind) and also controls many vital life processes (e.g., circulation, respiration, etc.). 'Ayama' signifies the voluntary effort to control and direct this prana. Breathing is one of the vital activities governed by prana on a gross level. This is the only pranic activity available to us, which can be regulated voluntarily. Secondly, the breathing system (pranic activity) is linked with the nervous system (base of the mental activity) on one hand and mind (consciousness) on the other.

Just like we have speed-breakers on the road to control the flow of traffic, we bring a 'pause' in breathing. So, pranayama means a voluntary and temporary pause in movement of the breath. From yogic point of view, it is a door between our physical existence and the spiritual path.

2. Science Behind Pranayam

Pranayam influences the autonomic nervous system, particularly the parasympathetic system, which promotes relaxation and counteracts the effects of stress. Deep and conscious breathing increases oxygen intake, improves lung capacity, and enhances the efficiency of the cardiovascular system. This physiological response triggers a relaxation response, reducing stress hormones like cortisol, lowering blood pressure, and calming the mind.

3. Benefits of Pranayam

1. **Reduce Stress and Anxiety:**Pranayam lowers cortisol levels, promoting a sense of calm and relaxation.
2. **Improve Respiratory Function:**Pranayam enhances lung capacityand increases oxygen supply to the body.
3. **Boost Immunity:** By increasing oxygen circulation and detoxifying the body, Pranayam strengthens the immune system, making it more effective in combating illnesses.
4. **Enhance Mental Clarity and Focus:** Controlled breathing techniques improve concentration, cognitive function, and memory thereby promoting mental clarity.
5. **Promote Emotional Stability:**Pranayam balances the Prana flow, leading to emotional equilibrium and resilience.

4. Few Pranayam Techniques

The practice of Pranayama is divided into three parts:

- Rechak (Exhalation)
- Purak (Inhalation) and
- Kumbhak (Retention of the breath).

These techniques are designed to cleanse the Nadis (energy channels), balance the Pancha Pranas, and awaken the subtle energies within the body.

1. **Nadi-Shodhan (Alternate Nostril Breathing):**It is known for its ability to harmonize the left and right hemispheres of the brain, promoting mental clarity and balance.
2. **Kapalabhati (Skull Shining Breath):** This technique is excellent for clearing nasal passages and improving lung function.
3. **Bhastrika (Bellows Breath):** It is often used to energize the body and prepare for meditation.
4. **Bhramari (Bee Breath):** This technique calms the nervous system, reduces stress, and helps alleviate anxiety and anger.
5. **Ujjayi (Ocean Breath):** It helps regulate body temperature, increases oxygen intake, and induces a state of relaxation.
6. **Sheetali and Sheetkari (Cooling Breath):** They cool the body, reduce anger, and lower blood pressure.

5. Role of Pranayam in Yoga and Meditation

Pranayam serves as a bridge between asana and meditation. In the practice of Yoga, asanas prepare the body by increasing flexibility and strength, while pranayam prepares the mind by calming the nervous system and focusing the attention. This makes it easier to enter a meditative state, where the mind becomes still, and deeper levels of consciousness can be accessed.Pranayamalso aids in the activation of the "Kundalini" energy, which is believed to lie dormant at the base of the spine. When awakened through specific Pranayam practices, this energy travels up the spine, through the chakras, leading to higher states of consciousness and spiritual awakening.

Understanding Pran and Pranayam is essential for anyone seeking holistic well-being and spiritual growth. Prana, as the vital life force, connects us to the universe, sustains our health, and nurtures our consciousness. Through the practice of Pranayam, we learn to harness this energy, leading to a balanced body, a focused mind, and a peaceful spirit.

5.

Types of Pranayama

Mrs. Arti Negi

Assistant professor

SGRRIM&HS ,

COLLEGE OF NURSING

Email: negiarti11@gmail.com

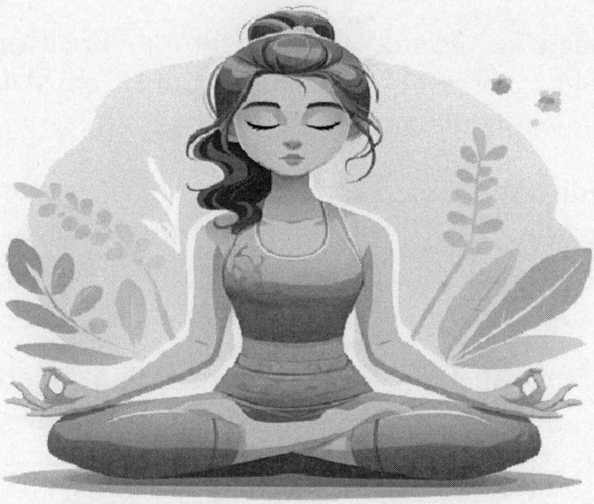

1. Introduction

Pranayama is a Sanskrit word that means "extension of the breath" or "breath control." It is a set of techniques used in yoga and Ayurveda to control and regulate the breath, promoting physical, mental, and spiritual well-being.

2. Types of Pranayama

There are several types of Pranayama, including:

1. **Ujjayi Pranayama** (Victorious Breath): A calming and balancing breath, characterized by a soft hissing sound.

2. **Kapalabhati Pranayama** (Breath of Fire): A rapid, forceful exhalation, followed by a passive inhalation.

3. **Bhastrika Pranayama** (Bellow's Breath): A rapid, forceful inhalation and exhalation, mimicking the movement of a bellows.

4. **Nadi Shodhana Pranayama** (Alternate Nostril Breathing): A balancing breath, where the practitioner alternates closing and opening the nostrils.

5. **Surya Bhedana Pranayama** (Sun Piercing Breath): A breath that stimulates the solar plexus, promoting energy and vitality.

6. **Chandra Bhedana Pranayama** (Moon Piercing Breath): A calming breath, that soothes the nervous system.

7. **Anuloma Viloma Pranayama** (Alternate Nostril Breathing with Retention): A variation of Nadi Shodhana, with breath retention.

8. **Bhramari Pranayama** (Bee Breath): A calming breath, that mimics the sound of a bee.

9. **Murcha Pranayama** (Swooning Breath): A breath that helps to relax and calm the nervous system.

10. **Kevala Kumbhaka Pranayama** (Retention of Breath): A breath where the practitioner holds their breath, without inhalation or exhalation.

3. Detailed Overview of each Pranayama including their Techniques and Benefits:

1. **Ujjayi Pranayama** (Victorious Breath):

Technique: Inhale and exhale through the nose, with a soft hissing sound.

Benefits: Calming, balancing, and relaxing.

2. **Kapalabhati Pranayama** (Breath of Fire):

Technique: Rapid, forceful exhalations, followed by passive inhalations.

Benefits: Stimulates digestion, energizes the body, and improves respiratory health.

3. **Bhastrika Pranayama** (Bellow's Breath):

Technique: Rapid, forceful inhalations and exhalations, mimicking a bellows.

Benefits: Stimulates the nervous system, improves respiratory health, and energizes the body.

4. Nadi Shodhana Pranayama (Alternate Nostril Breathing):

Technique: Close one nostril and inhale through the other, then switch to exhale through the other nostril.

Benefits: Balances the nervous system, improves respiratory health, and prepares for meditation.

5. Surya Bhedana Pranayama (Sun Piercing Breath):

Technique: Inhale through the right nostril, retain, and exhale through the left nostril.

Benefits: Stimulates the solar plexus, improves digestion, and boosts energy.

6. Chandra Bhedana Pranayama (Moon Piercing Breath):

Technique: Inhale through the left nostril, retain, and exhale through the right nostril.

Benefits: Calms the nervous system, improves respiratory health, and promotes relaxation.

7. Anuloma Viloma Pranayama (Alternate Nostril Breathing with Retention):

Technique: Alternate nostril breathing with breath retention.

Benefits: Balances the nervous system, improves respiratory health, and prepares for meditation.

8. Bhramari Pranayama (Bee Breath):

Technique: Inhale and exhale through the nose, making a humming sound like a bee.

Benefits: Calms the nervous system, improves respiratory health, and promotes relaxation.

9. Murcha Pranayama (Swooning Breath):

Technique: Inhale deeply, hold, and exhale slowly, feeling like you're going to swoon. Benefits: Relaxes the nervous system, improves respiratory health, and promotes relaxation.

10. Kevala Kumbhaka Pranayama (Retention of Breath):

Technique: Hold your breath without inhaling or exhaling.

Benefits: Improves respiratory health, increases oxygenation, and prepares for meditation.

4. Some Additional Pranayam

1. **Pranava Pranayama (Om Breath):** A calming breath, where the practitioner repeats the sound "Om" during inhalation and exhalation.

2. **Kumbhaka Pranayama (Breath Retention):** A breath where the practitioner holds their breath, without inhalation or exhalation.

3. **Sitali Pranayama (Cooling Breath):** A breath where the practitioner inhales through the mouth, and exhales through the nose.

4. **Sitkari Pranayama (Hissing Breath):** A breath where the practitioner inhales and exhales through the mouth, with a hissing sound.

5. **Bhaja Pranayama (Bellow's Breath):** A rapid, forceful inhalation and exhalation, mimicking the movement of a bellows.

6. **Surya Bhedana Kumbhaka:** A breath retention technique that stimulates the solar plexus and enhances energy.

7. **Chandra Bhedana Kumbhaka:** A breath retention technique that calms the nervous system and promotes relaxation.

8. **Uddiyana Bandha Kumbhaka:** A breath retention technique that engages the abdominal muscles and enhances core strength.

9. **Maha Bandha Kumbhaka:** A breath retention technique that engages all three bandhas (muscle locks) and promotes spiritual growth.

5. Benefits of Pranayam

a) Improves lung function and increases oxygen capacity.

b) Reduces symptoms of asthma and other respiratory disorders.

c) Enhances cardiovascular health and reduces blood pressure.

d) Supports immune function and overall health.

e) Improves mental clarity, focus, and concentration.

f) Reduces stress, anxiety, and depression.

g) Enhances overall well-being and quality of life.

h) Enhances spiritual growth and self-awareness.

i) Improves respiratory and cardiovascular health.

j) Increases oxygenation of the body.

k) Enhances mental clarity and focus.

l) Supports immune function and overall health.

m) Prepares for advanced meditation and yoga practices.

6. Conclusions

Each Pranayama has its unique benefits, and practitioners should approach them under the guidance of a qualified yoga or Ayurveda teacher. Remember to practice Pranayama under the guidance of a qualified yoga or Ayurveda teacher, especially if you're new to these techniques. They can help you choose the most appropriate Pranayama for your individual needs and abilities.

6

Yoga: The Art of Mindful Living

Rohini Chourasiya

Govt. Girls College, Vidisha

Email: rohinichourasiya2000@gmail.com

1. Introduction

Yoga is the oldest system of development encompassing body mind and spirit which has its origin goes back more than 5000 years ago. Yoga is a Sanskrit word for "union" means an experience of oneness or union with our inner being. This union is mind uniting with our body and breath to attain a higher level of consciousness. The integrated approach of mind and body control leads to ultimate physical health and happiness together with the achievement of mental peace and tranquility. In modern times, the value of yoga is being increasingly recognised for general health and its preventive and curative effects. Yoga is an ancient art based on a harmonising system for development of the body, mind and spirit. Yoga signifies the integration of personality at the highest level.

2. Yogasanas

Asanas are body positions in which one remains steady and comfortable both physically and mentally, for a desired length of time without strain. Asanas help the muscles relax by improving blood circulation which in turn relieves built up tension and stress. Stretching help to tone and condition the muscles and help as a therapy to prevent injuries.

Yoga breathing technique (Pranayama) is very powerful since they work as a tonic to reduce stress, insomnia, emotional balance, headache etc. "Prana" refers to vital air or energy and "Yama" is the control and direct of that energy "Pranayama" therefore is the control and direct of this vital energy via steady breathing the prana resulting in good heath.

Pranayama is the Sanskrit word meaning "extension of the prana or breath" or more accurately, "extension of the life force". The origin of this yogic discipline lies in ancient Bharat (India) or what is known as present day Hinduism Sanatan Dharm.

3. Limbs of Yoga

Maharishi Patanjali has defined yoga to have eight limbs like the part of the body namely,

1. Yam (Ethics)
2. Niyam (Rules)
3. Asan (Posture)
4. Pranayama (Breath)
5. Pratyahara (Withdrawing the senses)

6. Dharna (Focusing the mind)
7. Dhyan (Meditation)
8. Samadhi (Unconditional bliss)

Out of these eight limbs first five are called "Bahirang" that is relating to the physical part of the body and the last three are called "Antarang" that is relating to mind.

Yama and Niyama controls the yogi's passions and emotions and keep him in harmony with his fellow man. Asanas keep the body healthy and strong and in harmony with nature. Pranayama and Pratyahara teach the aspirant to regulate breathing and control the mind. Dharna, Dhyana and Samadhi take the yogi into the innermost recesses of his soul.

4. Branches of Yoga

The six branches of yoga are:

1. Hatha yoga (physical yoga)
2. Bhakti yoga (yoga of devotion)
3. Raja yoga (focuses on meditation and contemplation)
4. Jana yoga (yoga of mind)
5. Karma yoga (path of service)
6. Tantra yoga (path of rituals)

5. Benefits of Yogasanas:

Yoga is a mental, physical and spiritual practise which helps in attaining a great mind, body and soul. Stretching helps relax and tone the muscles to improve circulation to regain the vital force or energy, loss or gain weight, feel and look young and improve concentration. It cam relieve conditions like stress, back pain, allergy, headaches, high and low blood pressure, insomnia and depression.

Yoga does not need any costly equipment and materials as playground, gyms etc and can be practised throughout the year. It helps in efficient working of vital organs like heart, lungs endocrine glands, liver, pancreas and helps in maintaining a good balance between various functions in the body.

Yoga can be practised by anyone at any age with any physical condition depending on individual needs e.g. athletes and dancers can practise for restoring the energy and to improve stamina, housewives for regenerating the energy and to reduce fatigue, neuromuscular coordination etc. executives to give a break to the overload mind, children to control the wandering mind, muscle toning, to improve memory and concentration.

Yoga, therefore is for all ages from 5 years to as long as we live. It is very important to practise yoga with the full mind and in relax mood. Best time to practise yoga is either in the morning or in the evening. It should be practised on empty stomach.

Although yoga is thought and practised in different ways, Hatha yoga is a unique combination of asanas, pranayama and meditation and an approach to achieve perfect physical and mental health, happiness and tranquility.

5.1. Physical Benefits

- Improved efficiency of the lungs and cardiovascular system.
- Less oxygen requirement of the muscles.
- More efficient use of respiratory muscles.
- Less likelihood of breathing difficulties such as shortness of breath.
- Improved range of motion of joints.
- Improved coordination.
- Maintenance of bone density.
- Decreased risk of injury.
- Reduced likelihood of being overweight.

5.2. Psychological Benefits

- Increased sense of wellbeing.
- Increased selfesteem.
- Greater self-confidence.
- Decrease in craving for tobacco, food and alcohol.
- Greater ability to relax.
- Better quality sleep.
- Improved concentration.
- Reduced chance of depression.

6. Conclusions

Yoga is not just another form of exercise, but it is an approach to the inner well being of mankind. The purpose of yoga to create harmony in the physical, vital, mental, psychological and spiritual aspects of the human being. Be a yogin always, is the loving instruction of Lord Krishna. Convert life into yoga, so that you may ensure success in all the fields of activity. By regular practise, by using your presence of mind, skill and wisdom you can become yogins and enjoy happiness and peace, whatever be the circumstances and conditions in which you are placed.

7.

Meditation: A Gateway to Inner Peace and Clarity

CA Dinesh Agrawal

FCA, B.Com

Sikar, Rajasthan

Email: dineshca1988@gmail.com

1. Introduction

Meditation is a centuries-old practice that has been used across cultures to achieve mental clarity, emotional balance, and spiritual growth. At its core, meditation provides a systematic approach to quieting the mind, fostering awareness, and cultivating a sense of peace. In today's fast-paced world, meditation has gained significant attention for its potential benefits, not only for personal well-being but also for enhanced cognitive functioning and overall quality of life.

2. Defining Meditation

Meditation can be defined as a practice of focused attention and mindfulness that leads to a heightened state of awareness and deep mental clarity. It involves quieting the mind, observing one's thoughts without attachment, and achieving a sense of calmness and tranquility. Meditation is not confined to any particular religious or philosophical tradition; it has been practiced across cultures worldwide, often as a tool for spiritual growth, self-awareness, or personal healing. The core objective of meditation is to reach a state of stillness and clarity, enabling individuals to connect with their inner selves.

3. Historical Roots of Meditation

Meditation has a long and varied history, with its origins dating back thousands of years. In ancient India, meditation was an integral part of the spiritual practices of the Vedic tradition, which included mindfulness, concentration, and mantra repetition. The Buddha's teachings on meditation, which became a central tenet of Buddhism, emphasized the importance of meditation in achieving enlightenment and liberation from suffering.

In the West, meditation was not as prevalent until the 20th century when Eastern practices gained popularity. During this time, figures such as Swami Vivekananda, Maharishi Mahesh Yogi, and the Dalai Lama brought meditation to global attention, particularly in the context of stress reduction, well-being, and personal development.

Over the decades, meditation has become a widely adopted practice, used in therapeutic settings, by individuals seeking self-improvement, and even in corporate environments to improve focus and productivity.

4. Types of Meditation

There are various forms of meditation, each with its own distinct method and purpose. Some of the most commonly practiced techniques include:

1. **Mindfulness Meditation**: Rooted in Buddhist tradition, mindfulness meditation encourages individuals to focus on the present moment. Practitioners are taught to observe their thoughts, feelings, and bodily sensations without judgment or attachment.
2. **Transcendental Meditation (TM)**: Developed by Maharishi Mahesh Yogi, TM involves the repetition of a mantra to help quiet the mind and reach a state of restful alertness. TM is known for its stress-reduction benefits and its emphasis on inner peace.
3. **Loving-Kindness Meditation (Metta)**: This form of meditation focuses on developing compassion and love for oneself and others. It involves silently repeating phrases such as "May I be happy, may I be healthy" and extending these wishes to loved ones, acquaintances, and even those with whom one has conflicts.
4. **Zen Meditation (Zazen)**: A form of seated meditation from the Zen Buddhist tradition, Zazen focuses on breath awareness and the cultivation of presence. It is often practiced in silence, with the aim of transcending the limitations of the ego and reaching a state of pure awareness.

5. **Yoga Meditation**: Yoga integrates physical postures (asanas) with breath control (pranayama) to promote mental stillness. Meditation in yoga is typically practiced after the body has been relaxed and aligned through asanas, facilitating deeper focus and mindfulness.
6. **Guided Meditation**: In this form of meditation, a teacher or recording leads practitioners through a series of visualizations, body scans, or mindfulness exercises. It is particularly helpful for beginners or those seeking structured guidance in their practice.

5. Meditation and Mental Health

One of the most significant benefits of meditation is its impact on mental health. Over the years, scientific research has demonstrated that meditation can alleviate symptoms of anxiety, depression, and stress, among other mental health conditions. Meditation helps regulate the brain's response to stress, reduces the production of stress hormones such as cortisol, and enhances emotional regulation.

Several studies have shown that meditation can increase the thickness of the prefrontal cortex, the part of the brain responsible for executive functions such as decision-making, attention, and emotional regulation. Moreover, regular practice of meditation can decrease the size of the amygdala, the brain's emotional center, which is associated with fear and anxiety responses. This neuroplasticity leads to greater emotional balance, increased resilience to stress, and enhanced clarity of thought.

Mindfulness meditation, in particular, has been widely studied for its ability to improve emotional well-being. Research has shown that mindfulness meditation reduces rumination (repetitive, negative thinking) and improves self-compassion, both of which are linked to reduced symptoms of depression. Mindfulness also enhances emotional intelligence by increasing self-awareness and empathy.

6. Meditation for Clarity of Thought

Another key benefit of meditation is its ability to improve cognitive clarity. In a world filled with distractions, our minds often become cluttered with thoughts, worries, and external stimuli. Meditation offers a way to filter out the noise and regain focus and mental clarity. It helps individuals develop the capacity to observe their thoughts without becoming overwhelmed by them, thus leading to better decision-making, problem-solving, and creativity.

The practice of mindfulness meditation, for example, improves attentional control, allowing practitioners to focus their mental resources on tasks that require concentration. In addition, meditation enhances cognitive flexibility, making it easier for individuals to switch between tasks and adapt to new information. By regularly practicing meditation, individuals develop greater mental clarity, enabling them to approach challenges with a calm and clear mind.

7. Scientific Evidence Supporting Meditation

The scientific community has increasingly recognized meditation as a tool for enhancing mental and physical well-being. Numerous studies have shown that meditation can have a profound effect on reducing stress, improving attention, and promoting emotional health. The growing body of research on meditation has led to its incorporation into clinical psychology, with therapies such as Mindfulness-Based Stress Reduction (MBSR) and Mindfulness-Based Cognitive Therapy (MBCT) gaining popularity.

For example, a study published in *Psychological Science* found that individuals who practiced mindfulness meditation for just two weeks showed improvements in cognitive performance and the ability to sustain attention. Similarly, a study in *The Journal of Alternative and Complementary Medicine* found that individuals who practiced mindfulness meditation for eight weeks had reduced symptoms of depression and anxiety.

Other studies have explored the benefits of meditation for physical health. Meditation has been shown to lower blood pressure, improve sleep, and enhance immune system functioning. It has also been linked to a reduction in symptoms of chronic pain, as evidenced by research published in *The Journal of Pain*.

8. Meditation in the Modern World

In the context of modern society, meditation offers a respite from the constant demands of technology, social media, and work-related stress. The fast-paced nature of contemporary life can often leave individuals feeling overwhelmed, disconnected, and mentally fatigued. Meditation offers a powerful antidote to these challenges by providing a structured method for mental relaxation, focus, and self-awareness.

The increasing popularity of meditation in modern society is reflected in the rise of apps and online resources designed to make meditation more accessible. Platforms such as Headspace, Calm, and Insight Timer offer guided meditations, mindfulness exercises, and relaxation techniques to millions of users worldwide.

These digital tools have made meditation more inclusive, helping individuals incorporate the practice into their daily routines, regardless of their time constraints or experience level.

Moreover, the corporate world has embraced meditation as a tool for improving employee well-being and productivity. Many companies now offer mindfulness training and meditation breaks to help employees manage stress, improve focus, and enhance creativity. The incorporation of meditation into workplace culture reflects a growing recognition of its value in promoting mental clarity and emotional resilience.

9. Meditation and Spiritual Growth

While meditation is often associated with stress reduction and cognitive improvement, it also plays a central role in spiritual development. In many religious and spiritual traditions, meditation is a means of cultivating a deeper connection with the divine, the universe, or one's true self. For example, in Hinduism and Buddhism, meditation is used as a tool for self-realization and enlightenment, while in Christianity, contemplative prayer can be seen as a form of meditation aimed at drawing closer to God.

Meditation facilitates spiritual growth by fostering a sense of inner peace and connection to something greater than oneself. It encourages individuals to transcend the limitations of their ego and experience a sense of unity with the world around them. Through regular practice, meditators often report a greater sense of purpose, clarity, and alignment with their values and goals.

10. Conclusions

Meditation is a transformative practice that offers numerous benefits for mental, emotional, and spiritual well-being. It serves as a gateway to inner peace, mental clarity, and self-awareness. In a world filled with distractions and stress, meditation provides a valuable tool for quieting the mind, reducing anxiety, and improving focus. The growing body of scientific evidence supporting the efficacy of meditation further underscores its significance in modern life. As individuals continue to seek ways to navigate the challenges of contemporary society, meditation will undoubtedly remain an essential practice for achieving balance, clarity, and peace.

Incorporating meditation into daily life can lead to profound personal growth and transformation.

Whether used for stress reduction, cognitive enhancement, emotional regulation, or spiritual growth, meditation offers a path to a more peaceful and fulfilling life.

8.

The Role of Yoga in Modern Stress Management

Dr. Lok Mani Gupta

Homoeopathic Doctor

Gupta Homoeo Clinic, Kota Rajasthan

Email: drlokmanigupta@gmail.com

1. Introduction

In today's fast-paced and demanding world, stress has become an almost inevitable part of daily life. From the pressures of work, education, and social relationships to the constant stimuli of technology, modern society can be overwhelming. Stress, if left unmanaged, can lead to a variety of physical, mental, and emotional issues, including anxiety, depression, burnout, and cardiovascular diseases. As the global community grapples with this challenge, there is an increasing interest in finding sustainable, holistic approaches to stress management. Among these approaches, yoga has emerged as a powerful tool for combating stress and promoting overall well-being.

2. Understanding Stress in the Modern World

Stress is a natural physiological response to perceived threats or challenges, often referred to as the "fight-or-flight" response. This response, activated by the sympathetic nervous system, prepares the body to deal with immediate danger by increasing heart rate, blood pressure, and the release of stress hormones such as cortisol and adrenaline. While this response can be beneficial in acute situations, chronic stress—resulting from prolonged exposure to stressors—can lead to various negative health outcomes, including:

1. **Mental Health Issues**: Chronic stress can contribute to the development of anxiety, depression, and mood disorders. Stress is often accompanied by rumination, negative thinking patterns, and difficulty concentrating.
2. **Physical Health Problems**: Long-term stress has been linked to several cardiovascular conditions, such as hypertension, heart disease, and stroke. It can also contribute to digestive problems, autoimmune disorders, and chronic pain.
3. **Emotional Exhaustion**: Prolonged stress leads to emotional burnout, characterized by feelings of fatigue, detachment, and a diminished sense of accomplishment.

In response to the growing concerns about stress-related health issues, many people are turning to practices like yoga, which offers a holistic approach to stress management that addresses both the mind and body.

3. What Is Yoga?

Yoga is an ancient practice originating from India that aims to unite the body, mind, and spirit. It incorporates a variety of physical postures (asanas), breathwork techniques (pranayama), meditation, and ethical principles to achieve a state of balance and harmony. While yoga has deep spiritual roots, modern practitioners often approach it as a means of promoting physical fitness, mental clarity, emotional stability, and stress relief.

Yoga is not merely a physical exercise; it is a comprehensive system designed to create an integrated sense of well-being. The physical postures in yoga enhance flexibility, strength, and coordination, while breathwork (pranayama) helps regulate the body's energy and calm the nervous system. Meditation, another key component of yoga, fosters mindfulness and self-awareness, allowing individuals to detach from the stresses of everyday life and cultivate inner peace.

4. Components of Yoga in Stress Management

Yoga, in its entirety, provides multiple tools that can be employed to manage stress. Below are some of the key components of yoga that play a significant role in reducing stress:

1. **Asanas (Physical Postures)**: The practice of yoga postures involves stretching, strengthening, and aligning the body in various ways. These postures

not only promote physical health but also help release built-up tension in the body, which is often a physical manifestation of stress. Certain postures, such as forward bends, backbends, and inversions, are known to have calming effects on the nervous system, helping to reduce the physiological markers of stress, such as heart rate and blood pressure.

For example, poses like **Child's Pose (Balasana)**, **Corpse Pose (Savasana)**, and **Legs Up the Wall (Viparita Karani)** are often used at the end of a yoga practice to promote deep relaxation and restore the body to a state of equilibrium.

2. **Pranayama (Breath Control)**: Breath is a powerful tool for managing stress, and pranayama techniques involve conscious control of the breath to regulate the flow of prana (vital energy) in the body. Pranayama helps calm the autonomic nervous system, reducing the intensity of the "fight-or-flight" response and promoting relaxation.

   Some of the most effective pranayama techniques for stress management include:

   - **Nadi Shodhana (Alternate Nostril Breathing)**: Balances the left and right sides of the brain, calming the mind and reducing anxiety.
   - **Ujjayi (Victorious Breath)**: Encourages a slow, deep breath that induces a sense of calm and focuses the mind.
   - **Bhramari (Bee Breath)**: Involves creating a humming sound with the breath, which has a calming effect on the mind and reduces stress.

3. **Meditation**: Meditation in yoga is used to cultivate mindfulness, awareness, and emotional regulation. It allows individuals to step away from their busy thoughts and find a place of stillness within. By focusing on the present moment, meditation helps break the cycle of stress-induced rumination and anxiety.

   Meditation techniques often used in yoga include:

   - **Mindfulness Meditation**: Focuses on observing thoughts and feelings without judgment.

   - **Guided Visualization**: Involves imagining peaceful and calming scenarios to foster relaxation.

   - **Mantra Meditation**: Repeating a sound, word, or phrase to anchor the mind and reduce distractions.

4. **Mindfulness and Awareness**: Yoga encourages a deep connection to the present moment, fostering mindfulness. Mindfulness refers to the practice of paying attention to one's thoughts, emotions, and bodily sensations in a non-judgmental way. By cultivating mindfulness, yoga practitioners are able to observe their reactions to stress and develop healthier coping mechanisms. This awareness can help individuals respond to stressful situations with clarity and composure rather than reacting impulsively.

5. **Relaxation Techniques**: Relaxation techniques, such as **Yoga Nidra**, are used in yoga to induce a deep state of rest and rejuvenation. Yoga Nidra, also

known as “yogic sleep,” is a guided meditation practice that induces a state of deep relaxation while maintaining conscious awareness. This practice helps reduce stress by promoting physical and mental relaxation and allowing the body to restore its natural balance.

5. Physiological Effects of Yoga on Stress

The physiological effects of yoga on stress are well-documented. Research has shown that yoga has a direct impact on the body’s stress response system, including the nervous system and endocrine system. Some of the key physiological benefits of yoga in stress management include:

1. **Reduction in Cortisol Levels:**

   One of the key physiological effects of yoga on stress is the reduction in cortisol levels, which is the body's primary stress hormone. Cortisol is released by the adrenal glands during stressful situations and is part of the body's natural "fight-or-flight" response. While this response can be beneficial in acute stress, prolonged or chronic stress leads to elevated cortisol levels, which can negatively affect health by contributing to conditions such as anxiety, depression, high blood pressure, weakened immune function, and weight gain.

   Studies have shown that regular yoga practice can lower cortisol levels, helping to mitigate the harmful effects of chronic stress. By reducing cortisol, yoga promotes relaxation and helps restore the body's natural balance, supporting overall well-being and emotional stability.

2. **Activation of the Parasympathetic Nervous System**: Yoga promotes the activation of the parasympathetic nervous system, often referred to as the "rest and digest" system. This is the counterpart to the sympathetic nervous system, which is responsible for the "fight-or-flight" response. Through techniques such as deep breathing and relaxation poses, yoga induces a state of calmness, lowering heart rate, blood pressure, and reducing muscle tension. This activation helps to counterbalance the harmful effects of chronic stress and promotes recovery and relaxation.

3. **Improved Heart Rate Variability (HRV)**: Heart rate variability, which refers to the variation in time between heartbeats, is a key indicator of the body's ability to adapt to stress. Higher HRV is associated with greater resilience to stress and improved emotional regulation. Yoga has been shown to improve HRV, suggesting that it helps strengthen the body's ability to respond to stress in a healthy manner.

4. **Decreased Blood Pressure**: Yoga has been shown to have a significant effect on lowering blood pressure, especially in individuals who suffer from hypertension due to chronic stress. The combination of breath control, physical postures, and relaxation promotes vasodilation (widening of blood vessels) and enhances

circulation, which helps reduce blood pressure levels.

5. **Reduction in Muscle Tension**: Stress often leads to the build-up of muscle tension, particularly in the neck, shoulders, and back. Through the practice of physical postures and stretches, yoga helps release this tension, promoting relaxation and reducing discomfort associated with stress-related muscle tightness.

6. **Boosted Immune Function**: Chronic stress weakens the immune system, making individuals more susceptible to illness. Research has indicated that yoga can improve immune function by reducing stress hormones and increasing the activity of immune cells. Regular yoga practice has been linked to enhanced resistance to infections and improved overall health.

6. Scientific Evidence Supporting Yoga for Stress Management

Numerous studies have demonstrated the effectiveness of yoga as a tool for managing stress. Research spanning clinical settings, workplace environments, and general populations has shown that yoga can reduce stress, enhance well-being, and improve mental health outcomes.

1. **Clinical Studies**: A systematic review published in *The Journal of Alternative and Complementary Medicine* found that yoga is an effective intervention for reducing symptoms of anxiety,

depression, and stress. Studies included in the review highlighted that yoga practitioners showed improvements in emotional regulation, psychological resilience, and overall mental health. In particular, mindfulness-based yoga interventions have been shown to be as effective as traditional therapies such as cognitive behavioral therapy (CBT) for reducing stress and improving mood.

2. **Workplace Studies**: Several studies in workplace settings have demonstrated that incorporating yoga into daily routines can improve employee well-being and reduce stress. A study published in the *International Journal of Yoga* found that employees who participated in yoga-based stress reduction programs reported lower levels of stress, anxiety, and fatigue, while also showing improvements in job satisfaction and productivity.

3. **University and College Studies**: Research conducted among university students has shown that yoga can significantly reduce stress, particularly during high-pressure periods such as exams. A study published in *The Journal of Behavioral Health* found that students who practiced yoga for eight weeks experienced a reduction in perceived stress, anxiety, and depression, as well as improvements in self-esteem and emotional regulation.

4. **Chronic Stress and Mental Health**: For individuals suffering from chronic stress, yoga can be an important adjunctive therapy.

Research has demonstrated that yoga can alleviate symptoms of post-traumatic stress disorder (PTSD), generalized anxiety disorder (GAD), and major depressive disorder (MDD). A study published in *Frontiers in Psychiatry* found that yoga was particularly beneficial for individuals with high levels of psychological distress, helping them regain a sense of calm and emotional balance.

7. Yoga as a Preventative Measure for Stress

Yoga is not only an effective treatment for managing existing stress, but it also serves as a powerful preventative tool. Regular practice can enhance resilience to future stressors by cultivating greater self-awareness, mindfulness, and emotional stability. By incorporating yoga into daily life, individuals can build a foundation of strength, flexibility, and inner peace, which enables them to cope with stress more effectively.

1. **Building Resilience**: Yoga promotes a mindset of mindfulness and acceptance, helping practitioners become more resilient to the challenges and uncertainties of life. The practice encourages individuals to approach stressful situations with a calm, focused mind, reducing the likelihood of being overwhelmed by stress.

2. **Enhancing Emotional Regulation**: Through its emphasis on self-awareness and emotional balance, yoga helps individuals develop the capacity to regulate their emotions in the face of

stress. Yoga teaches individuals to observe their thoughts and emotions without becoming reactive or judgmental, fostering a greater sense of emotional control.

3. **Improving Focus and Clarity**: Yoga improves attention and mental clarity, which can help individuals navigate stressful situations with greater focus. Techniques such as breath awareness and meditation improve concentration and help individuals stay present, reducing the impact of stress on their mental state.
4. **Creating a Sustainable Lifestyle**: One of the most significant benefits of yoga is its ability to be seamlessly integrated into daily life. Unlike other stress management techniques that may require significant time or effort, yoga can be practiced in short bursts throughout the day. Even a brief session of yoga, such as a few minutes of deep breathing or a few simple postures, can help reduce stress and restore mental equilibrium.

8. Integrating Yoga into Daily Life for Stress Management

To fully experience the benefits of yoga for stress management, it is important to make it a regular part of one's routine. This can be done in a variety of ways:

1. **Morning Routine**: Starting the day with a short yoga session can set a positive tone for the day ahead. Simple stretches and breathing exercises

can help clear the mind, reduce tension, and increase energy levels, providing a strong foundation for managing stress throughout the day.

2. **Midday Breaks**: Taking a yoga break during lunch or a mid-afternoon slump can help reset the body and mind. Short sessions of deep breathing, stretching, or a quick relaxation pose can help reduce accumulated stress and improve focus for the remainder of the day.
3. **Evening Wind-Down**: Practicing yoga in the evening can help unwind from the stresses of the day. Relaxation techniques, such as Yoga Nidra or gentle stretches, promote deep relaxation and prepare the body for restful sleep, which is essential for managing stress and maintaining health.
4. **Yoga for the Workplace**: Incorporating yoga into the workplace through desk stretches, mindfulness techniques, or guided sessions can provide employees with effective tools for managing work-related stress. Employers can offer yoga programs or provide space for employees to practice during breaks to enhance overall well-being and productivity.

9. Conclusions

Yoga offers a powerful, holistic approach to stress management that addresses the mind, body, and spirit. Through its combination of physical postures, breath control, meditation, and mindfulness, yoga helps reduce the physiological and psychological effects of stress, fostering relaxation, emotional balance, and resilience. The scientific evidence supporting yoga's effectiveness in reducing stress, anxiety, and depression is robust, making it an invaluable tool in modern life. By incorporating yoga into daily routines, individuals can not only manage stress more effectively but also cultivate a deeper sense of well-being, clarity, and inner peace. In a world where stress is a common challenge, yoga provides a timeless and accessible solution for achieving a balanced and peaceful life.

9.

Yoga for Emotional Resilience and Mental Health: A Conceptual Paper

Anil Kuntal

Assistant professor,

FIITJEE Ltd., Delhi

Email: anilkuntal149@gmail.com

1. Introduction

In today's fast-paced and often stressful world, mental health challenges such as anxiety, depression, and emotional instability have become increasingly prevalent. The need for effective methods to enhance emotional resilience and mental well-being has never been more critical. Yoga, an ancient practice with deep philosophical and physical roots, has gained recognition as a powerful tool for fostering emotional resilience and promoting mental health. This conceptual paper explores how yoga serves as a transformative practice for emotional well-being, delving into its theoretical underpinnings, its evidence-based benefits, and its role in addressing various mental health challenges.

2. Understanding Emotional Resilience

Emotional resilience refers to the ability to adapt and recover from adversity, stress, and emotional setbacks. It involves managing emotions in a healthy manner, maintaining psychological stability, and bouncing back from challenges. Resilience does not imply the absence of stress or emotional discomfort, but rather the capacity to cope with and navigate difficult emotions, uncertainties, and life's inevitable difficulties.

Emotional resilience is critical for mental well-being as it enhances an individual's ability to manage stress, foster positive emotional states, and maintain a sense of inner peace even in the face of adversity. It is a key component of overall mental health and well-being, particularly in our modern society, where many people struggle to balance personal, social, and professional demands.

3. Yoga and Emotional Resilience: A Holistic Approach

Yoga is a holistic practice that integrates physical postures (asanas), breath control (pranayama), meditation, and mindfulness. Its foundational principles of balance, self-awareness, and mindfulness make it an ideal practice for enhancing emotional resilience. Through the consistent practice of yoga, individuals learn to develop a greater awareness of their emotional state, regulate their responses to stress, and cultivate inner strength.

Yoga encourages practitioners to observe their thoughts and emotions non-judgmentally, fostering emotional awareness and acceptance. The deep connection between mind and body in yoga practice enables individuals to process emotions, release emotional tension, and regulate their stress response.

4. The Science Behind Yoga for Emotional Resilience

Yoga's effectiveness in promoting emotional resilience is supported by a growing body of scientific evidence. Research across clinical, community, and workplace settings demonstrates that yoga has significant benefits for emotional health. Below, we explore the key scientific mechanisms through which yoga enhances emotional resilience.

4.1. Mindfulness and Emotional Awareness

At the heart of yoga is mindfulness—the practice of being fully present and aware of one's thoughts, feelings, and bodily sensations without judgment. This mindfulness approach allows individuals to build emotional awareness and recognize negative thought patterns or emotional responses before they escalate. Through yoga, individuals learn to cultivate a deeper understanding of their emotional triggers and develop the ability to respond consciously rather than react impulsively.

Mindfulness practices in yoga, such as focused breathing and meditation, train the mind to stay in the present moment. This helps break the cycle of rumination and excessive worrying, which are often associated with anxiety and depression. Research indicates that mindfulness-based practices in yoga can lead to significant improvements in emotional regulation, particularly by helping individuals manage negative emotions like anger, fear, and sadness.

4.2. The Regulation of the Autonomic Nervous System

Yoga has a profound effect on the autonomic nervous system (ANS), which regulates the body's involuntary functions, including heart rate, digestion, and stress responses. The two branches of the ANS—the sympathetic nervous system (SNS) and the parasympathetic nervous system (PNS)—work in opposition to one another. The SNS is responsible for the body's "fight-or-flight" stress response, while the PNS is responsible for "rest-and-digest" functions that promote relaxation.

Yoga practice, particularly pranayama (breathing exercises) and restorative postures, activates the PNS, promoting a state of relaxation. By stimulating the PNS and calming the SNS, yoga helps reduce the physiological markers of stress, such as elevated heart rate, high blood pressure, and increased muscle tension. This physiological relaxation contributes directly to emotional stability and resilience.

A study published in *Psychosomatic Medicine* found that yoga practitioners exhibited lower levels of cortisol (the stress hormone) and greater activation of the PNS, which contributed to improved emotional regulation and stress resilience.

4.3. The Role of Breath Control (Pranayama)

Breath control, or pranayama, is a key component of yoga that helps regulate both physical and emotional states. Slow, deep, and controlled breathing has been shown to reduce anxiety, stress, and emotional reactivity. Through pranayama, yoga practitioners learn to modulate their breath to induce a state of calm and focus, which aids in regulating emotions.

Research suggests that pranayama can activate the parasympathetic nervous system, leading to a reduction in heart rate and blood pressure, and promoting feelings of relaxation and emotional stability. In fact, pranayama has been shown to significantly lower cortisol levels, reduce anxiety, and improve mood regulation in individuals with stress-related disorders.

4.4. Yoga's Effect on Neurotransmitters and Brain Function

Yoga influences brain activity and neurochemistry, enhancing the brain's ability to regulate emotions. Neuroimaging studies have shown that yoga increases the volume of gray matter in areas of the brain involved in emotional regulation, such as the prefrontal cortex, hippocampus, and amygdala. The prefrontal cortex plays a key role in executive functions, including decision-making and emotional control, while the amygdala is associated with emotional responses, particularly fear and anxiety.

Yoga has also been shown to increase the production of neurotransmitters such as serotonin and gamma-aminobutyric acid (GABA), which are involved in regulating mood and anxiety. Higher levels of serotonin are associated with a positive mood and increased emotional resilience, while GABA promotes relaxation and reduces the effects of stress.

A study in *The Journal of Neuroscience* found that regular yoga practice resulted in increased gray matter density in the prefrontal cortex and hippocampus, areas associated with emotional regulation, cognitive flexibility, and resilience to stress.

4.5. Reduction of Negative Emotional States

Yoga has a direct impact on reducing negative emotional states such as anxiety, depression, and stress. Research consistently shows that yoga helps to reduce symptoms of depression and anxiety by promoting mindfulness, reducing negative self-talk, and enhancing emotional regulation. A meta-analysis published in *The Journal of Clinical Psychology* found that yoga was as effective as traditional therapeutic interventions, such as cognitive-behavioral therapy (CBT), in alleviating symptoms of anxiety and depression.

In particular, yoga provides an alternative to rumination—a common cognitive pattern in individuals with depression or anxiety. The practice encourages individuals to step away from negative thought cycles and focus on the present moment, fostering a sense of peace and emotional balance.

4.6. Building Emotional Resilience Through Self-Awareness and Acceptance

Yoga encourages self-awareness and self-acceptance, two key components of emotional resilience. Through consistent practice, individuals learn to be more attuned to their internal experiences, such as emotions, thoughts, and physical sensations. This self-awareness allows individuals to respond to challenges with greater emotional intelligence and less emotional reactivity.

Yoga also teaches self-acceptance by fostering an attitude of non-judgment and self-compassion. In yoga, there is no competition or need to achieve perfection—individuals are encouraged to accept themselves as they are. This mindset helps individuals build emotional resilience by reducing feelings of shame, self-doubt, and frustration, which often exacerbate stress and emotional struggles.

5. Yoga for Specific Mental Health Conditions

5.1. Yoga for Anxiety and Stress

Yoga has been widely studied for its effectiveness in reducing anxiety and stress. Practices such as gentle asanas, restorative yoga, and pranayama have been shown to significantly reduce anxiety symptoms and promote a sense of calm. A study published in *The Journal of Alternative and Complementary Medicine* found that yoga was highly effective in reducing perceived stress and anxiety in both healthy individuals and those with anxiety disorders.

5.2. Yoga for Depression

Yoga has been shown to be an effective adjunct to traditional treatments for depression. Regular yoga practice can help alleviate depressive symptoms by improving mood, reducing feelings of sadness, and enhancing self-esteem. A study published in *The*

American Journal of Psychiatry found that individuals who practiced yoga regularly experienced a significant reduction in depressive symptoms, particularly in combination with other forms of treatment.

5.3. Yoga for Trauma and PTSD

Yoga has been used as an effective therapeutic tool for individuals suffering from trauma and post-traumatic stress disorder (PTSD). The practice helps individuals reconnect with their bodies, release stored trauma, and regulate their emotions. Research has shown that trauma-sensitive yoga can significantly reduce symptoms of PTSD, including hypervigilance, emotional numbness, and intrusive thoughts.

6. Conclusions

Yoga is a transformative practice that offers a powerful and evidence-based approach to enhancing emotional resilience and mental health. Through its emphasis on mindfulness, breath control, emotional awareness, and physical postures, yoga fosters emotional regulation, reduces stress, and promotes a sense of well-being. The scientific evidence supporting yoga's impact on the brain, autonomic nervous system, and overall emotional resilience highlights its potential as a therapeutic tool for individuals struggling with anxiety, depression, and other mental health challenges.

By cultivating self-awareness, acceptance, and a sense of inner peace, yoga empowers individuals to respond to emotional challenges with greater resilience, clarity, and balance. As mental health concerns continue to rise in the modern world, yoga provides an accessible, holistic solution for enhancing emotional resilience and promoting long-term mental well-being.

10.

The Science behind Yoga: Evidence-Based Benefits

Saurabh Gupta

Assistant Manager

UCO Bank, Bijainagar

Email: saurabhwinner.gupta@gmail.com

1. Introduction

Yoga, an ancient practice originating from India, has evolved into a widely practiced discipline that transcends physical fitness, extending to mental, emotional, and spiritual well-being. Over recent decades, there has been an increasing body of scientific research examining the multifaceted benefits of yoga, with studies exploring its effects on physical health, mental well-being, and overall quality of life. These studies highlight the efficacy of yoga not only as a physical practice but also as a comprehensive therapeutic tool.

2. Yoga: An Overview

Yoga is a holistic discipline that involves physical postures (asanas), breath control (pranayama), meditation, and ethical principles aimed at fostering harmony between the body, mind, and spirit. While traditionally rooted in spiritual practices, yoga in the modern context is primarily practiced for its physical and mental health benefits, including improved flexibility, strength, relaxation, and stress reduction.

The practice of yoga encompasses different styles and forms, ranging from physically demanding styles such as Ashtanga and Vinyasa to more gentle practices such as Hatha and restorative yoga. Regardless of the style, all forms of yoga emphasize mindful breathing and focus on cultivating body awareness and self-regulation.

3. Scientific Evidence Supporting Yoga's Benefits

In recent years, a growing body of scientific evidence has emerged that substantiates yoga's many benefits. Research has consistently demonstrated that yoga is not only an effective stress management tool but also a significant contributor to physical health and mental well-being. The following sections explore the evidence-based benefits of yoga in greater detail.

3.1. Physiological Benefits of Yoga

Yoga is widely known for its positive effects on physical health. Numerous studies have highlighted the improvements in cardiovascular health, musculoskeletal function, and overall fitness that result from regular yoga practice. Some of the primary physiological benefits supported by scientific research include:

a. Improved Cardiovascular Health

Regular yoga practice has been shown to reduce risk factors associated with cardiovascular disease, such as high blood pressure, high cholesterol, and high heart rate. Studies indicate that yoga helps to lower systolic and diastolic blood pressure, particularly in individuals with hypertension. A review published in *The American Journal of Hypertension* found that yoga was associated with a significant reduction in both systolic and diastolic blood pressure in people with prehypertension and hypertension. This effect is likely due to the combined benefits of physical postures and breath control, which promote relaxation and reduce the body's stress response.

b. Enhanced Flexibility and Strength

Yoga is well-known for enhancing flexibility, especially in the spine, hips, and shoulders. The gradual stretching and lengthening of muscles help improve joint mobility and reduce the risk of injury. Additionally, many yoga postures require the use of body weight to build strength, which leads to increased muscle tone and endurance. Studies indicate that yoga can increase muscle strength, particularly in the core, arms, and legs, by engaging multiple muscle groups during asanas.

c. Pain Reduction

Yoga has been shown to be an effective intervention for chronic pain management. Research suggests that yoga can help alleviate conditions such as back pain, arthritis, migraines, and fibromyalgia. A study published in *The Journal of Pain* demonstrated that individuals with chronic low back pain who practiced yoga experienced significant reductions in pain intensity, improved mobility, and increased quality of life. The practice of yoga encourages body awareness and relaxation, which helps to alleviate tension and discomfort caused by physical pain.

d. Improved Respiratory Function

Pranayama, or controlled breathing, is a core component of yoga that plays a key role in improving respiratory function. Studies have shown that pranayama exercises increase lung capacity, improve oxygenation of the body, and enhance the efficiency of the respiratory system. For example, a study published in *The International Journal of Yoga* found that participants who practiced pranayama techniques exhibited improved pulmonary function and greater control over their breathing, which is particularly beneficial for individuals with asthma and chronic obstructive pulmonary disease (COPD).

3.2. Psychological and Emotional Benefits of Yoga

Yoga has long been praised for its ability to enhance mental and emotional well-being. Numerous studies have investigated the effects of yoga on conditions such as anxiety, depression, stress, and trauma. The evidence suggests that yoga has a positive impact on psychological health by reducing symptoms of mental health disorders and improving emotional regulation.

a. Stress Reduction

One of the most widely recognized benefits of yoga is its ability to reduce stress. Yoga helps to activate the parasympathetic nervous system, the body's "rest and digest" mode, which counters the effects of the sympathetic nervous system's "fight-or-flight" response. As a result, yoga reduces heart rate, blood pressure, and cortisol levels, leading to a sense of calm and relaxation. A meta-analysis published in *The Journal of Alternative and Complementary Medicine* concluded that yoga is an effective intervention for reducing perceived stress and promoting relaxation.

b. Reduction in Anxiety and Depression

Multiple studies have examined the effects of yoga on anxiety and depression, with promising results. Research published in *The Journal of Clinical Psychology* found that yoga was as effective as traditional therapies, such as cognitive behavioral therapy (CBT), in reducing symptoms of anxiety and depression. Yoga helps regulate the autonomic nervous system, promoting emotional balance and reducing the physiological markers of anxiety and depression, such as increased heart rate and muscle tension.

A study in *Psychosomatic Medicine* demonstrated that yoga significantly reduced symptoms of depression in individuals with major depressive disorder (MDD). The practice of mindfulness and meditation within yoga fosters self-awareness, encouraging individuals to observe their thoughts and emotions in a non-judgmental way, which can help break the cycle of negative thinking patterns associated with depression.

c. Improved Sleep Quality

Yoga has also been shown to improve sleep quality by promoting relaxation and reducing the physiological markers of stress. Studies indicate that individuals who practice yoga regularly experience deeper, more restful sleep. Research published in *The Journal of Alternative and Complementary Medicine* found that individuals with insomnia who practiced yoga experienced improvements in sleep duration, sleep quality, and overall well-being. The calming effects of yoga, particularly through relaxation poses and breathing techniques, contribute to the activation of the parasympathetic nervous system, helping individuals achieve restful sleep.

d. Enhanced Emotional Regulation

Yoga helps practitioners cultivate emotional regulation by increasing mindfulness and self-awareness. A study published in *Mindfulness* found that yoga practice leads to enhanced emotional regulation by encouraging individuals to observe their emotions without becoming overwhelmed by them. This ability to remain grounded in the present moment fosters resilience in the face of emotional stressors and promotes greater emotional stability.

3.3. Neurological Effects of Yoga

In addition to its physiological and psychological benefits, yoga also has profound effects on brain function and neuroplasticity. The practice of yoga, especially meditation and mindfulness, has been shown to enhance brain health, improve cognitive function, and increase emotional resilience.

a. Brain Structure and Function

Research suggests that yoga can enhance brain structure and function, particularly in areas related to emotional regulation, memory, and attention. Functional magnetic resonance imaging (fMRI) studies have shown that yoga practice increases gray matter density in regions of the brain such as the prefrontal cortex, hippocampus, and amygdala. These areas are involved in higher cognitive functions such as decision-making, memory, and emotional regulation.

A study published in *The Journal of Neuroscience* found that individuals who practiced yoga regularly had increased gray matter volume in the prefrontal cortex, a region associated with executive function and emotional control. This suggests that yoga may enhance cognitive flexibility, improve decision-making, and contribute to better emotional regulation.

b. Improvement in Focus and Attention

Yoga, particularly mindfulness and meditation practices, improves attention and concentration by training the mind to focus on the present moment. Studies have shown that individuals who practice yoga regularly exhibit better attention span, improved focus, and reduced cognitive fatigue. A study published in *Psychological Science* found that yoga practitioners performed better on tasks that required sustained attention and concentration compared to non-practitioners.

c. Neuroplasticity and Resilience

Yoga has been shown to enhance neuroplasticity, the brain's ability to reorganize and adapt to new experiences. This is particularly important for individuals coping with stress, trauma, or mental health disorders. By fostering neuroplasticity, yoga helps individuals build resilience to stress and trauma, allowing them to respond more adaptively to challenging situations.

3.4. Yoga for Disease Prevention and Management

Beyond its role in promoting general well-being, yoga is also a valuable tool in the prevention and management of various chronic diseases. Research has demonstrated the efficacy of yoga in improving outcomes for conditions such as cardiovascular disease, diabetes, arthritis, and chronic pain.

a. Cardiovascular Disease Prevention

Yoga has been shown to reduce the risk factors associated with cardiovascular disease, including high blood pressure, high cholesterol, and obesity. A study published in *The European Journal of Preventive Cardiology* found that individuals who practiced yoga regularly had a lower risk of cardiovascular events and improved heart health compared to non-practitioners.

b. Diabetes Management

Yoga can play a role in managing type 2 diabetes by improving blood sugar control, reducing inflammation, and promoting weight loss. Studies have shown that yoga helps lower fasting blood glucose levels, improve insulin sensitivity, and reduce the need for medication in individuals with type 2 diabetes.

c. Chronic Pain and Arthritis

Yoga has been shown to be effective in managing chronic pain, including conditions such as osteoarthritis, rheumatoid arthritis, and fibromyalgia. Regular yoga practice helps improve flexibility, reduce inflammation, and alleviate pain by increasing muscle strength and promoting relaxation.

4. Conclusions

Yoga is a powerful, evidence-based practice that offers a wide range of benefits for both physical and mental health. Research supports its efficacy in improving cardiovascular health, musculoskeletal function, stress management, and mental well-being. By enhancing flexibility, strength, and emotional regulation, yoga serves as a holistic tool for maintaining and improving health. Furthermore, yoga has demonstrated its potential in disease prevention and management, offering therapeutic benefits for chronic conditions such as cardiovascular disease, diabetes, and chronic pain. As scientific research continues to explore the benefits of yoga, it is clear that this ancient practice offers a wealth of health-promoting effects that can be integrated into modern wellness practices.

11.

Yoga for a Tranquil and Sustainable Future: A Comprehensive Path to Holistic Well-being

Minkal Tuteja

Panipat Institute of Engineering and Technology,

Samalkha Panipat, Haryana-132102

Email: drminkal.pharmacy@piet.co.in

Abstract

This paper explores the role of yoga as a transformative tool for fostering a peaceful and sustainable future, emphasizing its holistic approach to well-being. Rooted in ancient Indian philosophy, yoga transcends physical exercise, integrating mental, emotional, and spiritual dimensions to promote overall health. By addressing key components such as mindfulness, emotional regulation, and ethical living, yoga offers solutions to modern challenges related to mental health, environmental sustainability, and social harmony. The practice encourages balance between individual well-being and collective responsibility, advocating for ethical principles such as non-violenceand environmental stewardship. Through the lens of contemporary research, this paper examines the physiological, psychological, and societal benefits of yoga, highlighting its potential to contribute to global sustainability efforts by fostering inner peace, resilience, and community cohesion. The paper concludes that yoga, as a holistic lifestyle, can play a pivotal role in creating a more tranquil, sustainable, and harmonious world.

Keywords: Yoga, Sustainable life, Well-being, Inner peace

1. Introduction

Yoga, derived from the Sanskrit word "yuj," meaning union, symbolizes a general approach to harmonizing the body, mind, and spirit. At its core are the multifaceted principles of physical postures (asanas), breath control (pranayama), and meditation. Asanas, ranging from gentle stretches to more advanced poses, promote physical flexibility, strength, and balance. **Pranayama,** the art of controlled breathing, serves as a bridge between the physical and the mental, fostering a deep connection with the breath to calm the mind. **Meditation,** a cornerstone of Yoga, cultivates mindfulness and self-awareness, facilitating a profound sense of inner peace. Beyond the physical realm, Yoga encompasses ethical guidelines known as the Yamas and Niyamas, offering a moral and philosophical compass for virtuous living. The Yamas include principles such as non-violence (ahimsa) and truthfulness (satya), while the Niyamas encompass self-discipline (tapas) and contentment (santosha).Yoga provides a theoretical framework for understanding yoga beyond its physical practice, exploring its philosophical roots, psychological impacts, and role in modern healthcare and wellness. Thiscollection often emphases on how yoga, which originates from ancient Indian traditions, can be applied in various disciplines like health, psychology, education, and even management. Here is an overview of the types of conceptual discussions found in academic literature regarding yoga, focusing on its philosophy, psychological and physiological benefits, and modern applications.

2. Philosophical Foundations of Yoga

Conceptualization of yoga often begin by exploring the philosophical reinforcements of yoga, which is based on ancient Indian scriptures such as the **Yoga Sutras of Patanjali** and the **Bhagavad Gita**. Yoga is traditionally considered a spiritual and ethical discipline aimed at achieving **moksha** (liberation) and **samadhi** (self-realization).

In these papers, the **eight limbs of yoga** outlined in Patanjali's *Yoga Sutras* are frequently discussed:

1. **Yama** (ethical disciplines)
2. **Niyama** (personal observances)
3. **Asana** (postures)
4. **Pranayama** (breath control)
5. **Pratyahara** (withdrawal of the senses)
6. **Dharana** (concentration)
7. **Dhyana** (meditation)

8. **Samadhi** (state of unity)

Holistic Well-being: Yoga is not just a physical practice but a lifestyle that promotes holistic well-being through ethical living, self-discipline, and mental clarity.

Union of Mind and Body: Conceptual works focus on the idea of yoga as a union between the mind, body, and spirit, aiming to transcend the material world and reach higher states of consciousness.

3. Psychological and Emotional Benefits of Yoga

Yoga has gained significant attention in modern psychology as a therapeutic practice that fosters emotional regulation, stress management, and psychological well-being. Conceptualization on the **psychological mechanisms** through which yoga impacts mental health, such as mindfulness, emotional regulation, and resilience.

- **Mindfulness**: Yoga, through breath awareness and meditation, fosters mindfulness, defined as non-judgmental awareness of the present moment. This mindfulness reduces stress and anxiety by promoting a sense of calm and mental clarity.
- **Emotional Regulation**: Practicing yoga helps in regulating emotions by fostering awareness of bodily sensations and encouraging calmness, which can mitigate emotional reactivity and improve coping mechanisms.
- **Stress Reduction**: Research papers conceptualize how yoga, through practices such as **Pranayama**

(breathing techniques) and **Dhyana** (meditation), reduces the body's stress response by lowering cortisol levels and activating the parasympathetic nervous system.

4. Yoga in Healthcare and Therapy

Recent conceptual papers explore how yoga can be integrated into healthcare systems as a complementary and alternative medicine (CAM) practice. This section describes the role of yoga in **preventive healthcare** and its application in managing chronic conditions, pain, and mental health disorders.

- **Yoga as a Preventive Practice**: Yoga is conceptualized as a preventive healthcare practice that fosters physical fitness, stress resilience, and mental clarity. Regular practice of yoga has been linked to reduced risk of lifestyle diseases such as hypertension, diabetes, and heart disease.

- **Therapeutic Yoga**: Yoga therapy, tailored to individual needs, has been studied for its benefits in treating chronic conditions such as arthritis, lower back pain, and anxiety disorders. Literatureexplores yoga as an adjunct to conventional treatments, emphasizing its low-risk, holistic nature.

- **Mind-Body Medicine**: Yoga is increasingly being discussed within the context of mind-body medicine, which emphasizes the interplay between mental and physical health. This approach suggests that yoga can improve health outcomes by addressing both the physiological and psychological dimensions of illness.

5. Yoga and Modern Education

Some conceptual papers explore how yoga can be integrated into educational systems to promote cognitive development, focus, and emotional resilience in students. Yoga, with its emphasis on concentration and mindfulness, is considered a powerful tool for enhancing learning outcomes.

- **Cognitive Enhancement**: Yoga practices such as meditation and breath control are discussed for their ability to enhance focus, attention, and memory. These practices are believed to stimulate brain regions associated with executive functions, making them beneficial for students.
- **Emotional Resilience in Children and Adolescents**: Yoga in schools has been conceptualized as a method to enhance emotional resilience by teaching students' techniques for managing stress, anxiety, and peer pressure. It also promotes social-emotional learning (SEL), fostering empathy, self-awareness, and relationship skills.

6. Yoga in Management and Leadership

An emerging area of conceptual research focuses on the application of yoga principles in management, leadership, and organizational development. Drawing on the philosophical and ethical dimensions of yoga, these papers propose that yoga can foster mindful leadership, ethical decision-making, and improved well-being in the workplace.

- **Mindful Leadership**: Yoga teaches leaders to cultivate mindfulness, self-awareness, and emotional regulation, which are critical for making balanced and ethical decisions.

- **Stress Management in the Workplace**: Conceptual works suggest that incorporating yoga into corporate environments can improve stress management, reduce burnout, and enhance overall productivity by fostering a balanced approach to work and life.
- **Ethical Leadership**: The ethical principles (yamas and niyamas) of yoga are proposed as a framework for developing ethical leadership, focusing on values such as integrity, non-violence, and self-discipline in business practices.

7. Conclusions

This compilation on yoga bridge ancient philosophy with contemporary applications, offering a comprehensive understanding of how yoga can be integrated into various aspects of modern life. From healthcare and mental health to education and corporate management, yoga is increasingly recognized as a valuable tool for promoting holistic well-being and personal growth. These papers provide a rich theoretical foundation for the continued exploration of yoga's benefits and its potential to enhance both individual and societal health.

References

1. Bryant, E. F. (2009). *The Yoga Sūtras of Patañjali: A New Edition, Translation, and Commentary.* North Point Press.

2. Khalsa, S. B. S., & Butzer, B. (2016). *Yoga in school settings: A research review. Annals of the New York Academy of Sciences*, 1373(1), 45-55.

3. Woodyard, C. (2011). *Exploring the therapeutic effects of yoga and its ability to increase quality of life. International Journal of Yoga*, 4(2), 49-54.

4. Butzer, B., Bury, D., Telles, S., & Khalsa, S. B. S. (2016). *Implementing yoga within the school curriculum: A scientific rationale for improving social-emotional learning and positive student outcomes. Journal of Children's Services*, 11(1), 3-24.

5. Saraswati, S. S. (2009). *Yoga for the workplace: A conceptual framework for leadership and productivity. Journal of Management Development*, 28(8), 700-711.

6. Bryant, E. F. (2009). *The Yoga Sūtras of Patañjali: A New Edition, Translation, and Commentary*. North Point Press.

7. Miller, B. (2014). *Yoga Philosophy of Patañjali: Containing his Yoga Aphorisms with Vyasa's Commentary in Sanskrit*. Routledge.

8. Khalsa, S. B. S., & Butzer, B. (2016). *Yoga in school settings: A research review. Annals of the New York Academy of Sciences*, 1373(1), 45-55.

9. Streeter, C. C., et al. (2012). *Effects of yoga on the autonomic nervous system, gamma-aminobutyric-acid, and allostasis in epilepsy, depression, and post-traumatic stress disorder. Medical Hypotheses*, 78(5), 571-579.

10. Field, T. (2016). *Yoga research review. Complementary Therapies in Clinical Practice*, 24, 145-161.

11. Woodyard, C. (2011). *Exploring the therapeutic effects of yoga and its ability to increase quality of life. International Journal of Yoga*, 4(2), 49-54.

12. Butzer, B., Bury, D., Telles, S., & Khalsa, S. B. S. (2016). *Implementing yoga within the school curriculum: A scientific rationale for improving social-emotional learning and positive student outcomes. Journal of Children's Services*, 11(1), 3-24.

13. Serwacki, M. L., & Cook-Cottone, C. (2012). *Yoga in the schools: A systematic review of the literature. International Journal of Yoga Therapy*, 22(1), 101-109.

14. Saraswati, S. S. (2009). *Yoga for the workplace: A conceptual framework for leadership and productivity. Journal of Management Development*, 28(8), 700-711.

15. Pandey, A., & Gupta, R. K. (2008). *Spirituality in management: A review of contemporary and traditional thoughts and agenda for research. Global Business Review*, 9(1), 65-83.

12.

Yoga for Different Life Stages: From Childhood to Old Age

Dr. Khushboo Gupta

Assistant Professor

Trilok Singh TT College

Lakshmangarh, Sikar (Rajasthan)

Email: drkhushboogupta2017@gmail.com

1. Introduction

Yoga is a versatile and holistic practice that has been embraced by people across the globe for its physical, mental, and spiritual benefits. Its practices of physical postures (asanas), breathing techniques (pranayama), meditation, and mindfulness offer an integrated approach to well-being. While the core principles of yoga remain consistent, the way it is practiced can vary significantly depending on an individual's life stage. Yoga's adaptability makes it a suitable practice for people of all ages, from childhood to old age.

2. Yoga in Childhood: Foundation for Physical and Emotional Development

Childhood is a crucial period for the development of physical, mental, and emotional health. Yoga in childhood focuses on building strength, flexibility, balance, and concentration while also fostering emotional resilience and social skills. At this stage, yoga serves as a fun and engaging activity that encourages healthy habits, body awareness, and self-regulation.

1. **Physical Benefits for Children**

   In children, yoga helps to improve posture, balance, and coordination. Regular practice of yoga enhances muscle strength, flexibility, and joint mobility. As children grow, their bodies experience rapid changes, and yoga can help prevent musculoskeletal imbalances that may result from poor posture or sedentary behavior. The practice of yoga can also improve cardiovascular fitness, contributing to overall physical health.

2. **Emotional and Psychological Development**

   Yoga promotes emotional resilience in children by fostering self-awareness, mindfulness, and emotional regulation. As children learn to connect with their breath and body, they become more attuned to their emotions. Yoga teaches them to manage feelings such as frustration, anxiety, and stress in a non-reactive way. Additionally, yoga can be a powerful tool for addressing issues like hyperactivity, attention deficit disorders (ADHD), and emotional challenges that children may face in their formative years.

3. **Building Concentration and Focus**

   Yoga encourages concentration and mindfulness through practices like simple breathing exercises, meditative pauses, and engaging in specific poses. These exercises help children improve attention span, focus, and the ability to stay present, which translates into better performance in academics and other activities. By practicing yoga, children also develop a greater sense of self-control and discipline.

4. **4. Social and Interpersonal Skills**

   Group yoga classes offer an excellent opportunity for children to work together, fostering collaboration, respect, and empathy. Learning to follow instructions and share space with others enhances social interactions and the development of interpersonal skills. Children also learn patience and tolerance through yoga, as they understand that progress in yoga is personal and individual.

3. Yoga in Adolescence: Navigating Change and Cultivating Resilience

Adolescence is a critical stage of life characterized by rapid physical, emotional, and psychological changes. As teenagers navigate these changes, yoga can be an invaluable tool for maintaining balance, fostering emotional well-being, and developing coping strategies for stress.

1. **Managing Stress and Anxiety**

   Teenagers often face academic pressures, social challenges, and identity exploration, all of which can lead to high levels of stress and anxiety. Yoga helps adolescents cope with these stressors by providing a practice that promotes relaxation, reduces anxiety, and improves mood. Pranayama (breathing techniques), in particular, is effective in reducing the physical symptoms of anxiety, such as shallow breathing and rapid heart rate.

2. **Enhancing Emotional Regulation**

   During adolescence, emotional volatility is common, and teens may experience mood swings, anger, and frustration. Yoga fosters emotional regulation by encouraging mindfulness and self-reflection. Regular practice helps teens build emotional intelligence, allowing them to identify and express emotions more effectively and constructively. Yoga also teaches the importance of non-judgment and self-acceptance, helping teens develop a healthier self-image.

3. **Physical Benefits for Growing Bodies**

   Adolescence is a period of intense physical growth, and yoga can help address the physical demands of this phase. Regular practice improves flexibility, posture, and alignment, which are crucial for developing strong, well-balanced bodies. Yoga also helps prevent and alleviate growing pains, muscle stiffness, and tension, particularly in the back and neck, which can result from long hours of sitting at desks or engaging in physical activities like sports.

4. **Promoting Self-Confidence and Body Awareness**

   Yoga encourages body awareness, which is vital during the rapid changes that occur during adolescence. As teenagers become more aware of their physical and emotional sensations, they develop a deeper connection to themselves. Yoga fosters a positive body image by emphasizing strength, flexibility, and internal awareness over external appearance. This can help counteract the societal pressures that teens often face regarding body image.

4. Yoga in Adulthood: Strengthening Mind and Body

Adulthood is a time of personal growth, professional challenges, and family responsibilities. Yoga offers a powerful tool for managing the demands of work, relationships, and personal goals while promoting physical health, emotional balance, and mental clarity. Yoga practice in adulthood is crucial for maintaining vitality, reducing stress, and cultivating emotional resilience.

1. **Stress Management and Work-Life Balance**

   Yoga's ability to reduce stress is one of its most valuable benefits for adults. In the fast-paced, high-pressure environment of modern life, yoga provides a sanctuary for relaxation, mindfulness, and mental clarity. Practices such as restorative yoga, pranayama, and meditation help to release the physical and mental tension accumulated during the day, promoting a sense of calm and well-being. These practices help adults develop coping strategies for managing stress and improving overall quality of life.

2. **Physical Health and Injury Prevention**

   For adults, yoga helps prevent and alleviate the physical issues that arise due to sedentary lifestyles or repetitive physical activities. Office work, long hours of sitting, and strenuous physical labor can lead to muscle tightness, back pain, and poor posture. Yoga counteracts these issues by promoting flexibility, strengthening the core, and improving alignment. Additionally, yoga's emphasis on injury prevention through proper alignment and mindful movement is beneficial for maintaining long-term physical health.

3. **Mental Clarity and Emotional Balance**

   Yoga helps adults maintain mental clarity, focus, and emotional balance. Meditation and mindfulness practices help to sharpen concentration and reduce mental fatigue, making it easier for adults to navigate daily challenges and make decisions with clarity. Yoga also helps to balance the emotions, cultivating a sense of peace and resilience in the face of life's challenges, whether personal, familial, or professional.

4. **Relationship and Social Connections**

   Yoga can enhance relationships by promoting communication, compassion, and emotional awareness. By practicing mindfulness and developing emotional resilience, adults are better equipped to handle conflicts and manage emotions within relationships. Furthermore, joining a yoga community fosters social connections, helping individuals feel supported and connected to others who share similar values of health and wellness.

5. Yoga in Older Age: Maintaining Health and Longevity

As individuals enter older age, maintaining physical and emotional health becomes increasingly important. Yoga provides a safe and effective practice for seniors to stay active, improve flexibility, and manage age-related health issues. It offers not only physical benefits but also mental and emotional advantages, fostering overall well-being and longevity.

1. **Maintaining Mobility and Flexibility**

   As we age, the body's natural range of motion and flexibility often decrease. Regular yoga practice helps older adults maintain or improve joint mobility and muscle flexibility, reducing stiffness and promoting ease of movement. Yoga poses, particularly those that focus on stretching, gentle twists, and joint mobility, are excellent for maintaining flexibility and preventing the degeneration of muscles and connective tissues.

2. **Promoting Balance and Coordination**

   Falls and balance-related injuries are common concerns for older adults. Yoga can help improve balance and coordination by focusing on strengthening the core, improving proprioception (awareness of body position), and enhancing flexibility. Certain yoga postures, such as standing poses and balance-focused asanas, promote stability and improve coordination, reducing the risk of falls.

3. **Mental and Emotional Well-Being**

   Yoga is particularly beneficial for older adults in promoting mental clarity, emotional stability, and social well-being. Meditation, breathing exercises, and relaxation techniques help reduce the effects of stress, anxiety, and depression that may arise in later years. Yoga also encourages mindfulness and presence, which can combat feelings of loneliness or isolation, providing seniors with a sense of purpose and connection.

4. **Chronic Disease Management and Pain Relief**

   Yoga can help older adults manage chronic health conditions, such as arthritis, diabetes, and hypertension. Gentle yoga poses, combined with deep breathing, improve circulation, reduce inflammation, and relieve chronic pain. Furthermore, yoga's focus on relaxation and stress reduction can improve overall quality of life, helping seniors manage the mental and emotional challenges of living with chronic conditions.

6. Yoga Asanas for Different Life Stages: From Childhood to Old Age

Yoga asanas (postures) are one of the most integral components of yoga practice, offering numerous benefits for physical, mental, and emotional well-being. The types of asanas practiced can vary according to age, physical capacity, and individual needs.

6.1. Yoga Asanas for Childhood (Ages 3-12)

In childhood, yoga should focus on building strength, flexibility, and coordination, while also encouraging emotional regulation and focus. The practice should be playful, engaging, and simple to suit the attention span and development of children. These asanas also help children develop body awareness, concentration, and positive emotional health.

1. Tadasana (Mountain Pose)

- **Benefits:** Builds posture, balance, and body awareness.
- **How to Do:** Stand tall with feet together, arms by the sides, and palms facing forward. Engage the legs, lift the chest, and reach the arms overhead, keeping the palms facing each other.

- **Child-Friendly Tip:** Ask children to imagine they are standing like a tall tree, reaching for the sky.

2. Vrikshasana (Tree Pose)

- **Benefits:** Improves balance, concentration, and leg strength.
- **How to Do:** Stand tall, place the sole of one foot on the inner thigh or calf of the opposite leg (avoiding the knee), and balance. Bring the palms together in front of the chest or extend arms overhead.
- **Child-Friendly Tip:** Let children imagine they are a tree swaying in the wind, which makes it more fun and imaginative.

3. Baddha Konasana (Butterfly Pose)

- **Benefits:** Increases flexibility in the hips and groin.
- **How to Do:** Sit with the legs extended in front, bend the knees, and bring the soles of the feet together. Hold the feet with the hands and gently press the knees toward the floor.
- **Child-Friendly Tip:** Encourage children to flap their "butterfly wings" as they breathe deeply.

4. Bhujangasana (Cobra Pose)

- **Benefits:** Strengthens the back, arms, and shoulders; improves flexibility in the spine.
- **How to Do:** Lie face down, place the hands under the shoulders, and press into the palms to

lift the chest while keeping the elbows slightly bent.

- **Child-Friendly Tip:** Have children imagine they are snakes rising up from the ground.

5. Balasana (Child's Pose)

- **Benefits:** Relieves tension in the back and promotes relaxation.
- **How to Do:** Sit on the heels, fold forward, and rest the forehead on the mat, extending the arms in front or by the sides.
- **Child-Friendly Tip:** Let children imagine themselves as little "resting animals" or "baboons" curled up in a safe space.

6.2. Yoga Asanas for Adolescence (Ages 13-18)

Adolescence is a time of growth and change, making yoga important for maintaining balance, improving focus, and fostering emotional regulation. It can also help teens manage stress, anxiety, and the physical challenges of rapid growth and hormonal shifts.

1. Adho Mukha Svanasana (Downward-Facing Dog)

- **Benefits:** Strengthens the arms, legs, and core; stretches the back and hamstrings; improves blood circulation.
- **How to Do:** Start on hands and knees, lifting the hips toward the ceiling while pressing the heels toward the floor. Keep the hands shoulder-width apart and feet hip-width apart.

- **Teen-Friendly Tip:** Encourage teens to imagine themselves as a dog stretching after a nap, creating a light and fun approach.

2. Setu Bandhasana (Bridge Pose)

- **Benefits:** Opens the chest, strengthens the back and legs, and stimulates the thyroid.
- **How to Do:** Lie on the back with knees bent, feet flat on the floor, and arms by the sides. Press the feet into the ground and lift the hips toward the ceiling, creating a bridge shape with the body.
- **Teen-Friendly Tip:** Guide teens to imagine their body as a bridge connecting different parts of their lives, balancing emotions and energy.

3. Utkatasana (Chair Pose)

- **Benefits:** Strengthens the thighs, glutes, and back while improving balance.
- **How to Do:** Stand with feet hip-width apart, bend the knees, and squat down as if sitting in an imaginary chair, keeping the arms extended overhead.
- **Teen-Friendly Tip:** Encourage them to hold the pose for a few breaths, envisioning building strength and determination.

4. Virabhadrasana II (Warrior II Pose)

- **Benefits:** Strengthens the legs, opens the hips, and promotes focus and determination.

- **How to Do:** Stand with feet wide apart, turn one foot outward, bend the knee, and extend the arms parallel to the floor, palms facing down.
- **Teen-Friendly Tip:** Teens can imagine themselves as warriors overcoming challenges, giving the pose a sense of empowerment.

5. Nadi Shodhana (Alternate Nostril Breathing)

- **Benefits:** Calms the mind, improves focus, and balances the nervous system.
- **How to Do:** Sit comfortably, use the right thumb to close the right nostril, inhale through the left nostril, then close the left nostril with the right ring finger, and exhale through the right nostril. Alternate the process.
- **Teen-Friendly Tip:** This breathing exercise can be done during stressful times, helping to clear the mind before exams or social challenges.

6.3. Yoga Asanas for Adulthood (Ages 19-60)

In adulthood, yoga serves as an essential tool for managing stress, preventing injury, and maintaining overall health. Adults can use yoga to manage work-life balance, promote strength and flexibility, and alleviate the physical and mental strain that comes with daily responsibilities.

1. Trikonasana (Triangle Pose)

- **Benefits:** Stretches and strengthens the legs, hips, and spine while improving balance.

- **How to Do:** Stand with feet wide apart, extend the arms to the sides, and reach one hand down toward the foot while the other arm reaches upward, forming a triangle with the body.
- **Adult-Friendly Tip:** Focus on lengthening the spine and opening the chest to improve posture.

2. Anjaneyasana (Low Lunge)

- **Benefits:** Opens the hips and stretches the hip flexors; strengthens the legs and improves balance.
- **How to Do:** Step one foot forward and bend the knee, keeping the other leg extended behind. Reach the arms overhead or place them on the front thigh for support.
- **Adult-Friendly Tip:** This asana is excellent for releasing hip tension, often caused by long hours of sitting at a desk.

3. Marjaryasana-Bitilasana (Cat-Cow Pose)

- **Benefits:** Increases flexibility in the spine, improves posture, and reduces back pain.
- **How to Do:** Start on hands and knees. Inhale to arch the back (cow pose) and exhale to round the spine (cat pose), moving fluidly between the two.
- **Adult-Friendly Tip:** Use this as a gentle warm-up to improve spinal health and release any tension in the back.

4. Uttanasana (Forward Fold)

- **Benefits:** Stretches the hamstrings, calves, and spine, helping to alleviate tension in the back and neck.
- **How to Do:** Stand with feet hip-width apart, slowly hinge forward from the hips, and let the head and neck relax toward the floor.
- **Adult-Friendly Tip:** This pose is particularly beneficial for those who experience stiffness in the lower back or tension from sitting.

5. Savasana (Corpse Pose)

- **Benefits:** Deep relaxation and stress reduction, aids in mental clarity and emotional balance.
- **How to Do:** Lie flat on the back with arms by the sides, palms facing up. Focus on deep, slow breathing and allow the body to relax completely.
- **Adult-Friendly Tip:** Use Savasana at the end of a yoga session to fully relax and integrate the benefits of the practice.

6.4. Yoga Asanas for Older Adults (Ages 60+)

As people age, yoga can help improve mobility, prevent injury, and alleviate common age-related issues such as arthritis, osteoporosis, and limited flexibility. The focus is on gentle movements, breath awareness, and maintaining balance and flexibility.

1. Viparita Karani (Legs-Up-The-Wall Pose)

- **Benefits:** Reduces swelling in the legs, promotes relaxation, and improves circulation.

- **How to Do:** Lie on the back with the legs extended up against a wall, and rest the arms by the sides. This is a restorative pose that promotes relaxation.
- **Older Adult-Friendly Tip:** Excellent for relaxing after a long day, especially if standing or walking for extended periods.

2. Chair Pose (Utkatasana) Using a Chair

- **Benefits:** Builds strength in the thighs, hips, and back, helps improve posture and balance.
- **How to Do:** Sit in a chair with feet flat on the ground, hips-width apart. From there, press through the feet and engage the legs as if you are about to stand, but keep the seat. Hold for a few breaths.
- **Older Adult-Friendly Tip:** This adaptation provides the support of a chair, making it safer and more accessible.

3. Supta Baddha Konasana (Reclining Bound Angle Pose)

- **Benefits:** Opens the hips and groin, provides a relaxing stretch for the back and legs.
- **How to Do:** Lie on the back, bend the knees, and bring the soles of the feet together. Allow the knees to drop open to the sides.
- **Older Adult-Friendly Tip:** Place pillows or blankets under the knees to provide extra support and comfort.

4. Ardha Matsyendrasana (Seated Twist)

- **Benefits:** Improves spinal mobility, aids digestion, and reduces tension in the back and shoulders.
- **How to Do:** Sit tall with one leg extended and the other bent across. Twist the upper body toward the bent knee, placing the opposite arm on the knee and the other hand behind.
- **Older Adult-Friendly Tip:** This pose can be modified by using a chair for extra support and ensuring gentle, controlled movements.

5. Shavasana with Deep Breathing

- **Benefits:** Relieves stress, improves sleep quality, and promotes mental clarity and emotional calm.
- **How to Do:** Lie flat on the back, arms by the sides, palms facing up, and focus on deep, slow breathing. Stay in this position for several minutes, focusing on the breath and relaxing every part of the body.
- **Older Adult-Friendly Tip:** This is a restorative pose that is particularly helpful in managing the stresses of aging.

7. Conclusions

Yoga is a valuable practice that offers numerous benefits across all stages of life. By adapting yoga practices to meet the needs of different life stages, individuals can experience the transformative benefits of yoga at any age. From childhood to old age, yoga supports physical health, emotional well-being, and mental clarity. In childhood, yoga fosters physical strength, emotional regulation, and concentration. In adolescence, it helps manage stress, build resilience, and enhance self-awareness. In adulthood, yoga supports stress management, injury prevention, and emotional balance. Finally, in older age, yoga promotes mobility, balance, pain relief, and mental health.

Yoga is a versatile practice that can be adapted for people of all ages, from childhood to old age. By practicing age-appropriate asanas, individuals can improve their physical health, mental clarity, and emotional well-being. The benefits of yoga are vast and profound, promoting strength, flexibility, balance, and mindfulness, making it a valuable tool for lifelong health and happiness. Yoga's ability to cultivate mindfulness, resilience, and well-being makes it a timeless and essential practice for fostering health and longevity throughout the lifespan.

13.

Benefits of Yoga Before, During and After Pregnancy

Shivani Khare

(Home Science)

Government Girls Post Graduate College, Satna (M.P.)

Summary

Yoga is a form of exercise that can have both physical and mental benefits for a pregnant woman. Even better, it can be an ideal activity to do during the prenatal and postpartum period as you can start your postpartum yoga practice with a few asanas and then move on. If you are pregnant or have recently given birth to your baby, prenatal and postpartum yoga can help your body in many ways. Pre-pregnancy, during pregnancy or pre-natal and post-natal yoga Facilitating fitness routine before and after childbirth Mood swings, fatigue and body aches in pregnant women due to physical, mental and emotional changes there are too many. However, yoga can be a great medium to handle the changes that occur during pregnancy and the postpartum period.

1. Introduction

Through the presented article, if a pregnant woman wants to maintain her overall health or wants an easy delivery, or she is a new mother who wants to get back in shape and overcome anxiety, these pre-natal and post-natal yoga Asanas will definitely help him. All exercises are beneficial for a healthy pregnancy. And even though it's safe to continue doing what you were doing before you got pregnant — like running, sailing or riding a Peloton bike — you may be looking for a low-impact way to exercise and minimize the side effects of pregnancy. . Enter. Prenatal yoga, a type of yoga that helps you connect with yourself and your baby during pregnancy. Whether you're new to yoga, there's a prenatal yoga practice for everyone.

2. Benefits of Yoga before, during and after pregnancy

Exercising regularly has many health benefits, the same applies to pregnant women and new mothers who are interested in doing prenatal and postpartum yoga . Even if you don't feel like getting up and doing yoga sometimes (which is totally normal), remember that the benefits in the long run far outweigh a few moments of rest.

Pregnancy requires a lot of physical and mental strength, so exercising before conception can help you in countless ways. After all, what could be better than preparing your body to safely carry a fetus for nine months.

3. Benefits of pre-pregnancy planning

- By doing yoga before pregnancy, your body gets prepared for the necessary energy for delivery.
- Furthermore, it is also related to increasing fertility and increasing the chances of safe and easy conception.

- Yoga before pregnancy makes you more emotionally stable by reducing stress and anxiety, thus preparing you for the psychological and emotional challenges during and after pregnancy.
- Most importantly, doing yoga before pregnancy increases muscle endurance and flexibility, which is essential for easy and simple delivery.

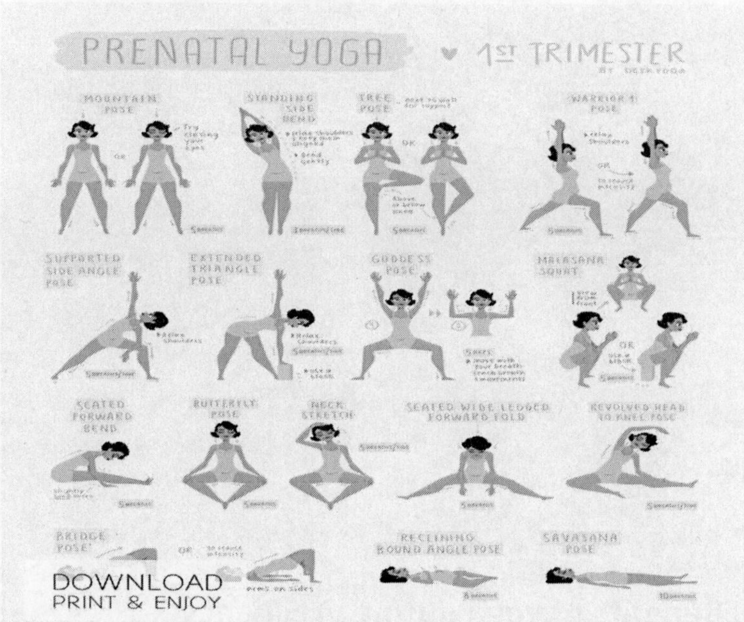

4. Yoga during pregnancy

A physically active woman delivers in less time and easier than a woman who was not so active during pregnancy. Although prenatal yoga postures are quite safe, please consult your gynecologist or midwife before starting any yoga routine. Even if your doctor allows it, make sure not to push yourself too hard and make sure your baby adjusts to his new routine slowly and comfortably.

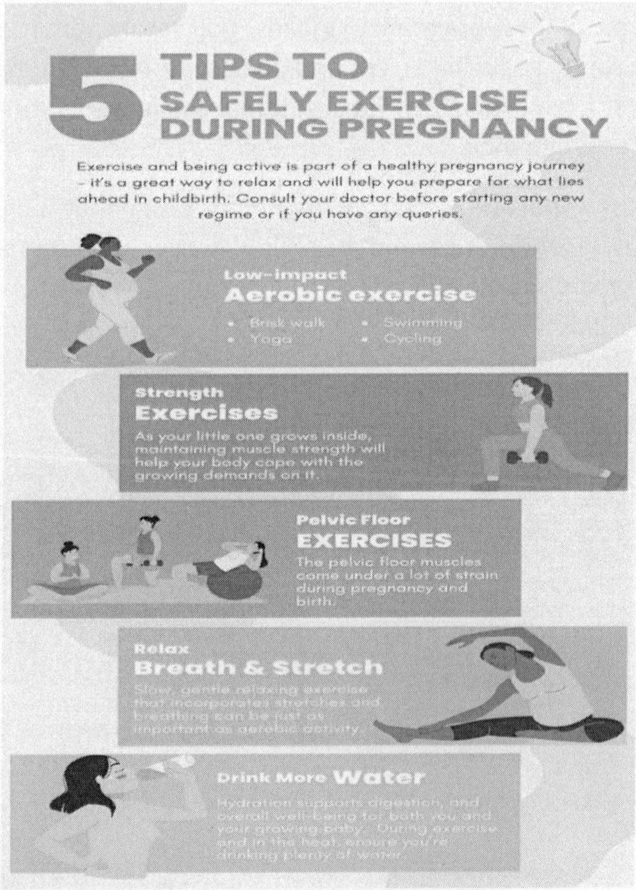
5 TIPS TO SAFELY EXERCISE DURING PREGNANCY
Exercise and being active is part of a healthy pregnancy journey – it's a great way to relax and will help you prepare for what lies ahead in childbirth. Consult your doctor before starting any new regime or if you have any queries.
Low-impact
Aerobic exercise
• Brisk walk
• Swimming
• Yoga
• Cycling
Strength
Exercises
As your little one grows inside, maintaining muscle strength will help your body cope with the growing demands on it.
Pelvic Floor
EXERCISES
The pelvic floor muscles come under a lot of strain during pregnancy and birth.
Relax
Breath & Stretch
Slow, gentle relaxing exercise that incorporates stretches and breathing can be just as important as aerobic activity.
Drink More Water
Hydration supports digestion, and overall well-being for both you and your growing baby. During exercise and in the heat, ensure you're drinking plenty of water.

5. Benefits of yoga during pregnancy

- Doing yoga during pregnancy helps in reducing back pain and swelling.
- It is also helpful in providing relief from constipation and preventing excess weight gain.
- Doing yoga during pregnancy helps you sleep better and increases energy levels.

- Yoga during pregnancy also prepares you for mental postpartum challenges by reducing stress and also keeps your mood stable.
- Most importantly, yoga during pregnancy trains your muscles and strengthens them for safe delivery and speedy recovery.

6. Postpartum Yoga

Women who have had an uncomplicated pregnancy and a normal delivery can start doing postnatal yoga a week after giving birth or as soon as they feel ready. However, if you have had a cesarean delivery or have any complications, please talk to your doctor to determine the time frame to know the right time to start yoga after pregnancy. Generally, most women are advised to wait until six weeks after giving birth.

7. Benefits of yoga after delivery

- Doing postpartum yoga with your baby can speed up his recovery and reduce pain.
- Postnatal yoga practice is helpful in strengthening muscles and reducing fat.
- Postpartum yoga can also improve your mental health, helping to deal with postpartum depression and difficulty socializing.
- It also helps in increasing your energy levels, balancing hormonal balance and reducing fatigue.
- Postpartum yoga asanas prevent lower back pain and stretch the abdominal muscles as well as strengthen loose ligaments and joints.

8. Safety Tips/Precautions for Pregnancy, Prenatal and Postpartum Yoga

- Always discuss with your doctor before starting prenatal or postpartum yoga.
- If you have never done yoga or exercise before, start with walking during pregnancy and gradually incorporate yoga during pregnancy and then start yoga after your doctor's approval.
- To be extra safe and to make sure you are doing it correctly to reap its benefits, always do prenatal or postpartum yoga under the guidance of a professional yoga instructor.
- Even if you are very comfortable with the recommended yoga postures, do not push yourself beyond your limits.
- Drink adequate amount of water, practice yoga in a well-ventilated room and protect your body from overheating.
- Do not do excessive stretching or vigorous yoga asanas.

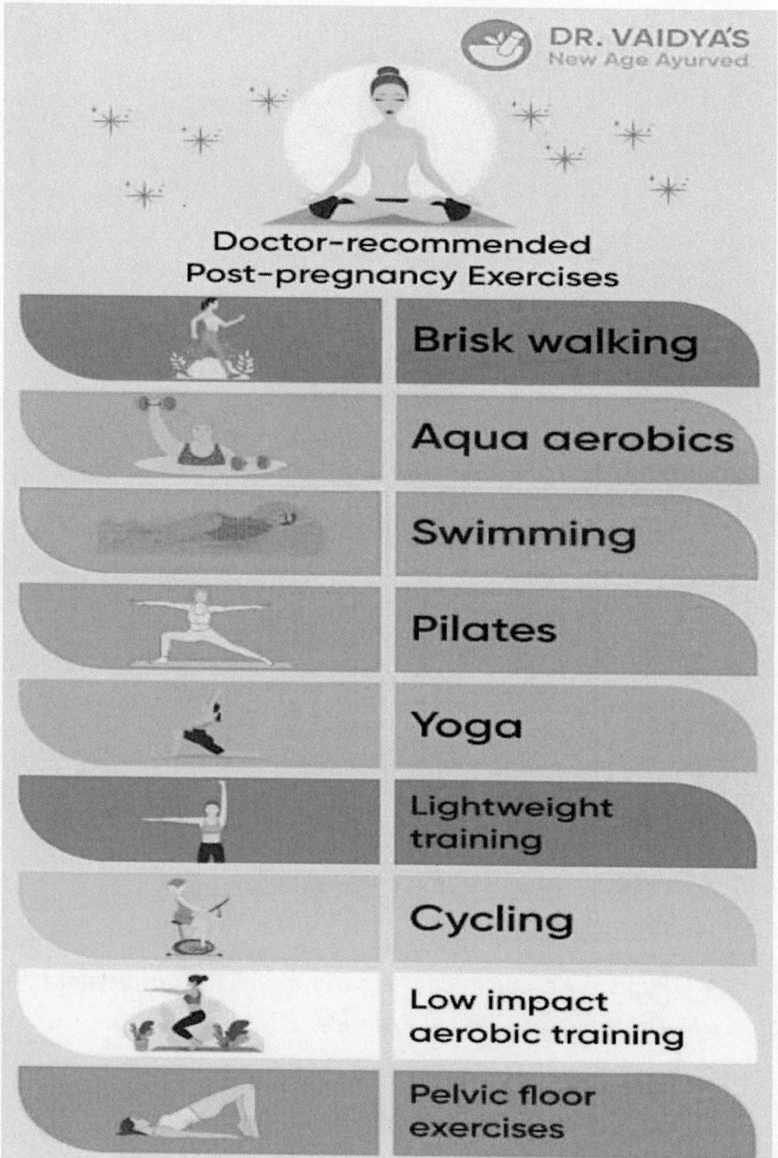
DR. VAIDYA'S
New Age Ayurved
Doctor-recommended
Post-pregnancy Exercises
Brisk walking
Aqua aerobics
Swimming
Pilates
Yoga
Lightweight training
Cycling
Low impact aerobic training
Pelvic floor exercises

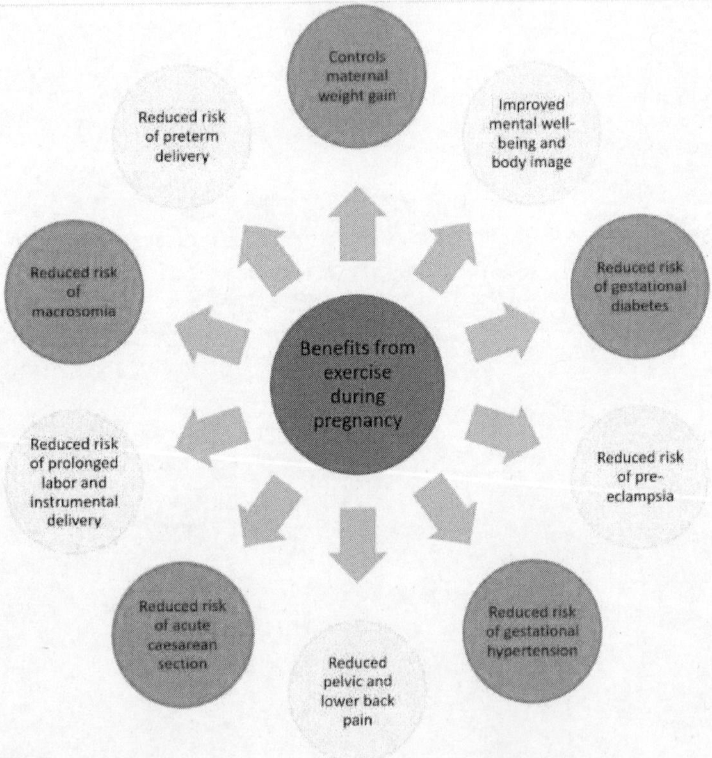

Bibliography

- https://www.webmd.com/baby/benefits-yoga-during-pregnancy
- Field T. Yoga clinical research review. *Complementary Therapies in Clinical Practice.* 2011;17(1):1–8.
- Wren AA, Wright MA, Carson JW, Keefe FJ. Yoga for persistent pain: new findings and directions for an ancient practice. *Pain.* 2011;152(3):477–480.
- Salmon P, Lush E, Jablonski M, Sephton SE. Yoga and mindfulness: clinical aspects of an ancient mind/body

practice. *Cognitive and Behavioral Practice.* 2009;16(1):59–72.

- Beddoe AE, Lee KA. Mind-Body interventions during pregnancy. *Journal of Obstetric, Gynecologic, and Neonatal Nursing.* 2008;37(2):165–175.
- Sandman CA, Davis EP, Buss C, Glynn LM. Prenatal programming of human neurological function. *International Journal of Peptides.* 2011;2011:9 pages.837596.

14.

Yoga during Pregnancy

Jyoti Dahiya

Self-Financing Guest Scholar

(Home Science Department)

Government Girls Post Graduate College, Satna (M.P.)

Email: jytsingh1303@gmail.com

Summary

Every woman has to go through many new experiences during pregnancy. It is very important for the mother to remain healthy for the proper development of the fetus. Any kind of carelessness during pregnancy can be harmful for the mother as well as the child in the womb. In this state, there is a need to take special care of the body. At this time, it is very important for women to remain physically as well as mentally healthy. Doctors advise pregnant women to take care of their diet and also do light exercise. Many hormonal changes also take place in the body at this time. Due to which many times the mind becomes disturbed or the body feels uncomfortable. For this, pregnant women should do some easy yoga asana every day. These yoga asana are very beneficial in improving the physical health as well as mental health of pregnant women.

1. Introduction

Yoga is an age-old traditional practice. It provides mental, physical, emotional and spiritual benefits. By doing yoga regularly, the body remains healthy. Doing yoga even during pregnancy is very beneficial for pregnant women. Doing pre-natal yoga does not cause much pain at the time of delivery. Some women also have pain in the stomach, waist etc. during pregnancy. Weight increases more. In such a situation, you can stay away from all these problems by doing yoga. Prenatal yoga is very healthy. Yogic techniques include asana, pranayama and meditation. Yoga reduces anxiety and helps women remain mentally calm during pregnancy. Yoga is a gentle form of exercise to stay fit and connect with your own body and baby during pregnancy.

2. Yoga during Pregnancy

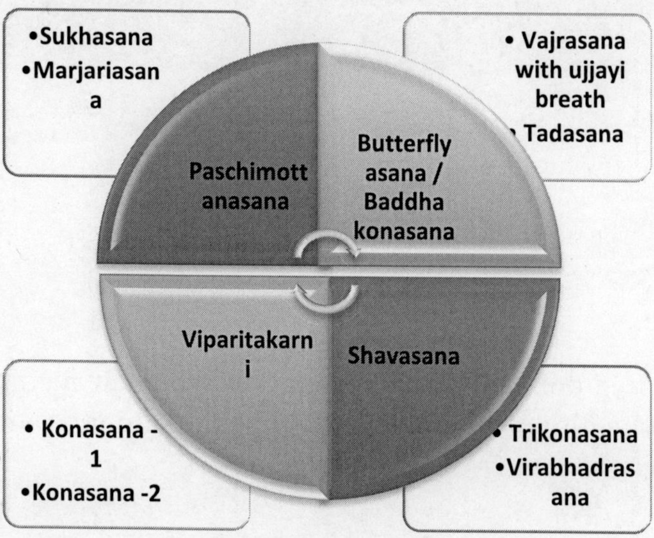

Doing asanas, pranayam and meditation during pregnancy is beneficial. This maintains peace in the mind. Maintain restraint during pregnancy. Yoga is a relaxing exercise to stay in shape during pregnancy and connect with the baby. It is suitable for everyone.

3. Some pranayams which can be done during pregnancy

- Ujjayi breath
- Full yogic breath
- **Bhramari Pranayama**
- Yoga nidra
- Nadi Shodhan Pranayam

After doing all these pranayam, you can meditate for some time which will give you complete relaxation.

4. Some precautions that should be taken during pregnancy

- If you are in the initial months of pregnancy, then do not do such asanas which are difficult and put more pressure on the lower abdomen.
- Some standing yoga asanas should be done during the first three months of pregnancy because it strengthens the muscles of the legs, provides good blood circulation in the body, provides energy and also removes stiffness and swelling in the legs. We do.
- During the middle three months of pregnancy, tiring, vigorous asanas should not be done. During the intervening three months, more time should be spent on pranayam and meditation.
- No yoga asana should be done from 10th to 14th week of pregnancy because this time is the most important time of pregnancy.
- Do not put too much pressure on your lower abdomen. Make sure that you do such yoga asanas that strengthen your shoulders and upper waist.
- There is no need for you to do every asana during pregnancy. Make sure you do only as much as you can comfortably.

5. Some yoga asanas which should not be done during pregnancy

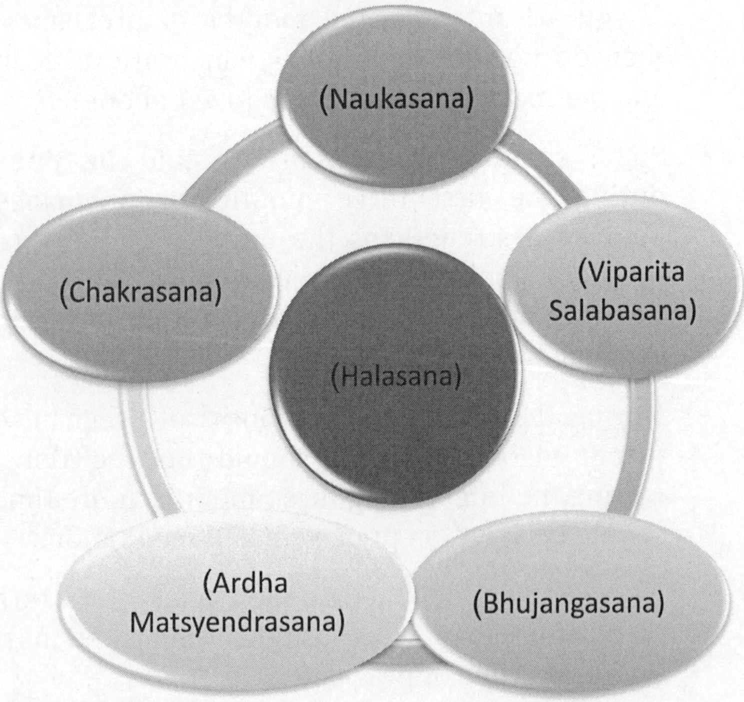

All yoga asanas involve breathing. There are some simple asanas that can be done during pregnancy, but still powerful. Practicing yoga daily during pregnancy keeps you healthy and also helps in keeping the mind and body focused during delivery. Doing yoga daily keeps your body active and also prevents common problems during pregnancy like constipation and vomiting. Doing yoga daily removes stress from the body, which increases the chances of a comfortable delivery. The tension is released from the uterus, fallopian tubes and pelvic area, due to which there is no problem in delivery. The Yogasanas given in the presented article which can be done during pregnancy, the above written Yogasanas protect you from the problems occurring during pregnancy and also assure a comfortable delivery. If a pregnant woman practices asanas daily, it does not take much time to recover after delivery.

Yoga practice has special importance during pregnancy. It is considered beneficial not only for the pregnant mother, but it also has many benefits for the baby in the womb. Practicing yoga during pregnancy strengthens the muscles and helps in preparing for delivery. Yoga also plays an important role in reducing mental stress. Doing yoga during pregnancy is safe, provided it is done under the guidance of a trained yoga guru.

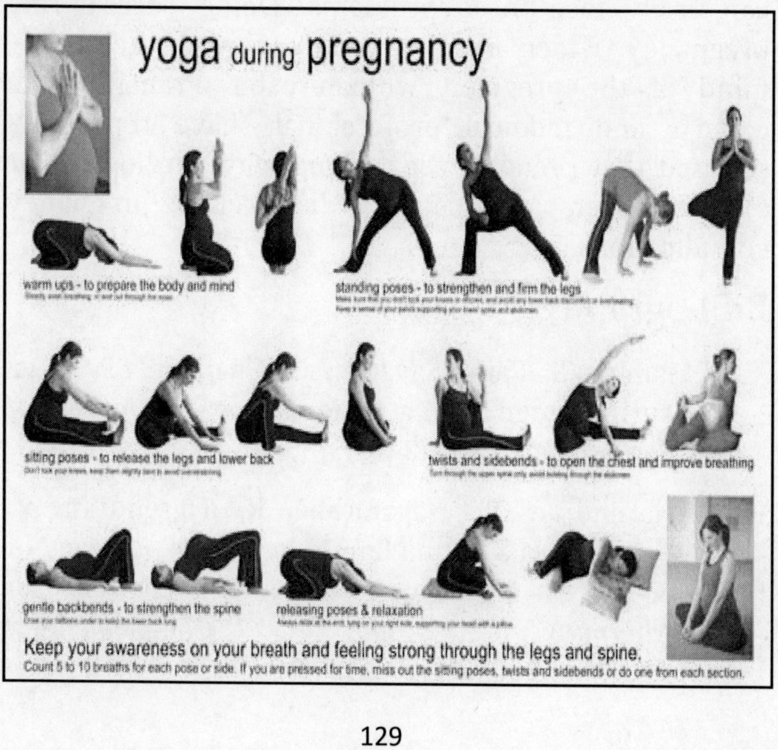

yoga during pregnancy
warm ups - to prepare the body and mind
standing poses - to strengthen and firm the legs
sitting poses - to release the legs and lower back
twists and sidebends - to open the chest and improve breathing
gentle backbends - to strengthen the spine
releasing poses & relaxation
Keep your awareness on your breath and feeling strong through the legs and spine.
Count 5 to 10 breaths for each pose or side. If you are pressed for time, miss out the sitting poses, twists and sidebends or do one from each section.

Yoga exercises are also very popular among pregnant women. But yoga during pregnancy is different from the commonly practiced yoga asanas. Prenatal yoga includes asanas and postures that are considered safe for pregnant women to practice. These asanas help stretch and tone the muscles that face the most pressure during pregnancy. They also help prepare you for labor and delivery.

Pregnancy is the most special time for any woman in which she feels happiness, hope and curiosity. The physically healthy and emotionally strong woman has a direct impact on the physical, mental and psychological development of the child. Fluctuations in a woman's mood, fatigue, leg pain, cramps and respiratory problems are a part of pregnancy, but pregnant women can easily face these problems. Doing yoga during pregnancy, which is called pre-natal yoga, keeps the mind of the pregnant woman calm. Prenatal yoga experts and medical professionals have repeatedly stressed that prenatal yoga, along with cardiovascular exercises such as walking, can help relieve pregnancy complications.

Bibliography

- Babbar S, Parks-Savage AC, Chauhan SP. Yoga during pregnancy: a review. *American Journal of Perinatology*. 2012;29(6):459–464.
- Narendran S, Nagarathna R, Narendran V, Gunasheela S, Rama Rao Nagendra H. Efficacy of yoga on pregnancy outcome. *Journal of Alternative and Complementary Medicine*. 2005;11(2):237–244.

- Rakhshani A, Maharana S, Raghuram N, Nagendra HR, Venkatram P. Effects of integrated yoga on quality of life and interpersonal relationship of pregnant women. *Quality of Life Research.* 2010;19(10):1447–1455.
- Satyapriya M, Nagendra HR, Nagarathna R, Padmalatha V. Effect of integrated yoga on stress and heart rate variability in pregnant women. *International Journal of Gynecology and Obstetrics.* 2009;104(3):218–222.
- Sibbritt D, Adams J, van der Riet P. The prevalence and characteristics of young and mid-age women who use yoga and meditation: results of a nationally representative survey of 19,209 Australian women. *Complementary Therapies in Medicine.* 2011;19(2):71–77.
- www.Nualawoulfe.ie
- www.mayoclinic.org

15.

Embracing Motherhood: The Transformative Power of Prenatal and Postnatal Yoga

Dr. Amrita Singh

Assistant Professor

Department of Home Science, IGNTU Amarkantak

Email: amrita.singh@igntu.ac.in

1. Introduction

Motherhood is a profound journey that encompasses physical, emotional, and spiritual transformations. As expectant mothers and new parents navigate this life-changing experience, prenatal and postnatal yoga have emerged as invaluable tools to support and empower them. The journey of motherhood begins with pregnancy, followed by childbirth, lactation, and nurturing. While the Collins dictionary defines 'a mother as a female who has given birth to offspring, the term also encompasses individuals who embody maternal affection and care.'

Prenatal and postnatal yoga have gained significant attention in recent years due to their numerous benefits for expectant mothers and new parents. Like a gentle embrace, these practices envelop women in a sense of comfort and empowerment, alleviating the aches and pains of pregnancy, while nurturing the body, mind, and spirit. As the journey progresses, prenatal yoga prepares the body for the miracle of childbirth, strengthening the muscles, and cultivating relaxation and stress relief techniques, while postnatal yoga tenderly supports the transition into motherhood, fostering a deeper connection between mother and child. With each breath, each movement, and each moment of stillness, prenatal and postnatal yoga weave a tapestry of wellness, resilience, and joy, empowering women to embrace the beauty and wonder of motherhood with confidence, grace, and love.

2. Prenatal Yoga: Empowering Expectant Mothers

As a woman's body blossoms with new life, pregnancy unfolds a complex tapestry of physical, mental, emotional, and intellectual transformations. Like a gentle rain soothing the earth, yoga tenderly prepares the expectant mother to navigate the challenges that arise during this remarkable journey. As happiness and stress entwine like the threads of a rich brocade, yoga offers a serene refuge, calming the mind and nurturing the spirit.

Pregnancy is a metamorphic odyssey, where a woman's inner and outer worlds undergo profound changes. Like a lotus blooming in the depths of a serene lake, she evolves, yet faces obstacles that ripple the surface of her daily life. As a pregnant woman embraces the ancient wisdom of yoga, she unlocks a treasure trove of benefits for herself and her unborn child. With each deliberate breath, she cultivates neuro-muscular control, harmonizing the coordinated relaxation and contraction of her uterus.

Ayurvedic and yogic texts reveal a plethora of asanas, tailored specifically for pregnant women, which consume minimal energy while yielding profound benefits. A wealth of scientific studies and published articles substantiate the transformative power of yoga during pregnancy, mitigating complications such as pregnancy-induced hypertension, intrauterine growth retardation, and pre-term delivery. Prenatal yoga is a modified practice tailored to meet the unique needs of expectant mothers. By embracing prenatal yoga, women can:

- Develop physical strength and flexibility, enhancing their ability to cope with pregnancy and childbirth.
- Cultivate emotional resilience, reducing stress and anxiety.
- Foster a deeper connection with their body and baby, promoting a sense of empowerment and confidence.

3. Asanas (postures) in prenatal yoga

1st trimester	2nd trimester	3rd trimester
Ardha Kati Chakrasana	Supta Badha Konasana	Moolabandha and Ashwini Mudra in Baddhakonasana

Chatushpadasana / Kriya	Balasana / Nikunja Asana	Chatus Pada Asana & Kriya
Trikonasana	Moolabandha	Vyagraha Pranayama
Vyagraha Pranayama / Chiri Kriya	Meruasana	Kukkriya Pranayama
Nikunja / Balasana	Badhakonasana	Bhramari Pranayama
Eka / Dwi Pada Uttana Asana	Jatraparivritha Asana	
Aswini Mudra	Navasana	
Baddhakona Asana / Kriya	Aswini Mudra	
Pranava Pranayama	Savitri Pranayama	
Moolabandha		

Studies have shown that prenatal yoga can lead to improved birth outcomes, reduced symptoms of depression and anxiety, and enhanced foetal well-being.With each deliberate breath, each mindful movement, and each serene moment of stillness, she crafts a rich tapestry of holistic wellness, resilience, and joy, welcoming the miracle of motherhood with open arms, confidence, and unconditional love.

4. Postnatal Yoga: Empowering New Mothers

The first month after giving birth is a time to recuperate and adjust. From 6 to 8 weeks postpartum, post-natal yoga is a great way to regain strength and stamina after giving birth and can easily include baby.Pregnancy and childbirth are physiologically tough for the body. During pregnancy, abdominal muscles are pushed out to the side to make room for baby, and baby's weight add pressure on women's pelvic floor, legs and feet.Postnatal yoga is a nurturing and restorative practice designed to support new mothers in their journey towards physical and emotional recovery after childbirth.

5. Asanas (postures) in Postnatal yoga

- Baddhakona Asana / Kriya
- Uddiyana Bandha
- Chatushpadasana / Kriya
- Eka / Dwi Pada Uttana asana
- Vyagraha Pranayama / Chiri Kriya
- Navasana
- Pavan Mukta Kriya

- Aswini Mudra
- Pranava Pranayama
- Moolabandha
- Shavasana with Savitri Pranayama
- Surya Pranayama

This gentle and low-intensity practice focuses on:

- Soothing stretches to release tension in areas tightened by caring for a newborn, such as the neck, shoulders, and back.
- Conscious breathing exercises to calm the mind, promote relaxation, and reconnect with your inner self.
- Gentle core exercises to strengthen and stabilize the abdominal muscles, improving posture and reducing the risk of injury.
- Pelvic floor engagement activities to restore tone and resilience, supporting bladder control and overall pelvic health.

This practice is typically modified to accommodate the unique needs and limitations of new mothers, making it accessible and beneficial for all. By embracing postnatal yoga, women can nurture their bodies, minds, and spirits, embracing the transformative journey of motherhood with greater ease, confidence, and joy.

6. Conclusions

Prenatal and postnatal yoga offer a transformative journey of empowerment for expectant mothers and new parents. By embracing these practices, individuals can cultivate physical, emotional, and spiritual resilience, leading to a more confident and empowered experience of motherhood. As we continue to explore the benefits of prenatal and postnatal yoga, it is essential to recognize their value in supporting maternal and foetal well-being.

In conclusion, incorporating yoga into pregnancy care offers a multitude of benefits for both mother and child, leading to a healthier and more empowered pregnancy journey. By integrating yoga into their pregnancy regime, women can attain a higher level of physical, mental, and emotional fitness, setting the stage for a positive and transformative birth experience. As a holistic practice, yoga supports the well-being of both mother and child, making it an invaluable addition to prenatal care. Embracing yoga during pregnancy can have a lasting impact on the health and happiness of the entire family, making it a wise and loving choice for expectant mothers.

List of Published Books

1. Gupta K and Jain M. Vridhopayogi Vyanjan: Vridhjano ke liye Upcharatmak Pak Vidhiyan. Abhinav Prakashan. Ajmer. 2016. ISBN: 978-938418946-4

This book contains more than 65 healthy food recipes developed, prepared and clinically verified by myself alone, tailored with the nutritional needs of the geriatric population.

2. Gupta K. Community Science and Sustainable Community Development. Lambart Academic Publication. Germany 2021. ISBN: 978-620419757-9

This book provides excellent research data related to different aspects of community which will be helpful to strengthen the sustainability of a community in terms of health, nutrition, wellness and economy.

3. Gupta K. 75 years of Indian Independence: Food and Nutritional Achievements, Opportunities and Challenges (Volume 1). Notion Press. Chennai. 2022. ISBN: 979-888883053-6

4. Gupta K. 75 years of Indian Independence: Food and Nutritional Achievements, Opportunities and Challenges (Volume 2). Notion Press. Chennai. 2022. ISBN: 979-888883757-3

5. Gupta K. 75 years of Indian Independence: Food and Nutritional Achievements, Opportunities and Challenges (Volume 3). Notion Press. Chennai. 2022. ISBN: 979-888909005-2

These three books provide enriched research data pertaining to various aspects of health, lifestyle, tourism, agriculture, antenatal or post natal diet, nutritional status, cognition and nutrition, etc., that will be extremely helpful to improve quality of life of the individuals ultimately making healthy and sustainable community.

6. Gupta K. Aazadi ka Amrit Mahotsav: Community Science Achievements, Opportunities and Challenges. BlueRose One Publishers. India. 2023. ISBN: 978-935704938-2

This book is particularly based on different disciplines of community science, i.e., food science and nutrition, food security, advancement in food preservation and processing, sustainable breeding and cultivation approaches in agriculture, importance of prebiotics, role of therapeutic diet, importance of nutrition for pregnant ladies and children, how cognitive development is affected by nutritional status of the children, spiritual development, skill based learning system DEASA, effect of social media on community development.

7. Gupta K. Nutrition Education: An Important Pillar of Health. Notion Press. Chennai. 2023. ISBN: 979-888959915-9

This book is particularly based on different topics of nutrition science, i.e., importance of nutrition in daily life, flavours of Bengal, flavours of Ramadan, Indian spices, celebrate a world of flavours, nutrition in bed bound patients, why nutrition is essential and importance of homemade pickles in daily diet.

8. Gupta K, Bhushan V, Pandey A. Issues with Girls. Notion Press. Chennai. 2023. ISBN: 979-889026221-9

This book is particularly based on different topics related to girls and women, i.e., change in education to bring empowerment, mental hygiene, health and diet management, rise in health problems: A wake up call, girls hygiene and nutrients, letting the girls grow naturally, nutrition for girls, optimal nutrition, good health and wellbeing,: are we there yet?, women's leadership and role model for girls, empowering girls: dare to dream, baby girl: beautiful miracles.

9. Gupta K, Tripathi KM, Meena N, Sukhwal I, Soni V. Recent Trends in Community Science. BlueRose One Publishers. India. 2023. ISBN: 978-935819026-7

This book is based on different area of community science, i.e., parenting techniques and changes in parenting over the time, association between eating out and childhood obesity, rural participation and community development, ergonomics for everyone, kitchen ergonomics, use of unconventional fibres in textile industry, sustainable techniques for dye application (textile industry), spiritual development, therapeutic nutrition, impact of dietary habits on people suffering from polycystic ovarian syndrome (PCOS), millets: heritage of India, *terminalia arjuna* herb and its impact on hypercholesterolemia's patients, black cumin seeds, development disorders of children and homoeopathic treatment, success stories of women entrepreneurs from fields of community science.

10. Gupta K, Katiyar P, Meena S, Tripathi KM,. Millets: The Miracle of Nature. Notion Press. Chennai. 2023. ISBN: 979-889066606-2

This book is particularly based on topics such as millets- the nutria-cereal, magical grains, millets- the climate resilient nutria cereals, India's treasury: millets as dietary accessory, therapeutic role of millets in daily life, nutritional impact of millets on pregnant mothers, economic aspects of millets etc,.

11. Gupta K, Cherian B, Ramalakshmi, Harjai K. Health and Wellness (A basic guide to obtain good health). Notion Press. Chennai. 2023. ISBN: 979-889067222-3

Chapters of this book entitled "Health and Wellness (A basic guide to obtain good health)" particularly based on topics such as Blood, breathing & thoughts, Meditation, yoga, silence and prayer, Mind-body connection: Using yoga to enhance maternal health, Improve your low self-esteem with blessings of yoga and meditation, Food habits, Nutrition for health, Biogreens: the immunity booster, Role of nutrition in obesity, No health without mental health, Ayurveda for holistic health care, Homoeopathic biochemic treatment, Palliative care, Functional foods in cardiovascular disease, Union government initiatives to provide affordable, accessible, and quality healthcare for all.

12. Gupta K, Gaur V, Kumari R, Mishra S, Arya L, Mukharjee G. Health for All. Notion Press. Chennai. 2023. ISBN: 979-889133024-5

The edited book volume is primarily intended to be a collection of peer reviewed and plagiarism free chapters written by research scholars, academicians, scientists, doctors and faculty members of their respective fields. Chapters of this book entitled "Health for All" particularly based on topics such as sustainable innovation strategies in public health, application of technology in healthcare, world health organization's policies on world nutrition, the invisible threat of food borne diseases, obesity in affluent societies and its effect, role of nutrition education, treatment of diseases using different medical systems, non communicable diseases through workplace wellness initiatives, immunization program and serum banking in India.

13. Gupta K, Swamy D, Jain S, Sangeeta, Rochani C, Verma R. Current Advances in Community Science. Notion Press. Chennai. 2023. ISBN: 979-889186087-2

The edited book volume is primarily intended to be a collection of peer reviewed and plagiarism free chapters particularly based on topics such as impact and benefits of nano-fertilizers, understanding the benefits of dietary fibres on health, importance of food fortification, consumer problems and protection in India related to adulteration, black marketing, health and psychological well-being, role of millets to sustain food and nutritional security, extension education in modern era, paradigm shift in extension approaches for sustainable development, computer aided designing in textiles and apparel industry, use of microfibers, Instagram as a tool to promote micro apparels and qualitative analysis on the different areas of skill development in community science.

14. Gupta K, Katiyar P, Verma P, Pawar RV, Sangeeta. Food Safety & Security- A Basic Guide. Notion Press. Chennai. 2023. ISBN: 979-889233007-7

Chapters of this book entitled "Food safety and food security (A basic guide)" particularly based on topics such as foodborne diseases, immunity boosters, feeding the nation, when food turns foul, national and international organizations working for food safety, food spoilage, food poisoning, food preservation, food safety, food security, food safety and standard authority of India (FSSAI), natural farming, food standards, food safety risk assessment and management, role of government in ensuring food safety, role of food pickles in achieving household food security, assessing the benefits and costs of improving food safety.

15. Gupta K, Venkatappa KG, Devi KV, Sangeeta, Pal P. Brain: Associations, Wellness & Treatment. Notion Press. Chennai. 2024. ISBN: 979-889233671-0

Chapters of this book entitled **"Brain: Associations, Wellness and Treatment"** particularly based on topics such as brain health and disabilities, what I learnt about our brain, heads off to migraine, effect of stress on mental health, unlocking mental wellness, Parkinson's disease and its homeopathic treatment, mental health, depression, interrelation between brain health and cognitive functioning, artificial intelligence and cognitive science, effect of sleep patterns on brain health, prioritizing brain health, spirituality and brain health, impact of financial condition on brain heath, drugs and brain health; and impact of homemade food on maintaining brain health and wellness.

16. Gupta K, Mukharjee G, Esaivani KB, Sangeeta, Anuradha K, Jethwani P. Handbook on Inflammatory Bowel Disease (Volume 1). Hemakshee Publication. Sikar. 2024. ISBN: 978-81-969920-0-2

This book titled **"Handbook on Inflammatory Bowel Disease (Volume 1)"** is primarily intended to be a collection of peer reviewed and plagiarism free chapters written by research scholars, academicians, scientists, doctors and faculty members of their respective fields. Chapters of this book particularly based on topics such as etiology differential diagnosis, prevention and treatment of inflammatory bowel disease (IBD); malnutrition and IBD, role of yoga & meditation in IBD, yoga techniques & quality of life in patients with IBD, role of diet in IBD, use of micro-organisms in prevention & treatment of IBD, role of remission diet in IBD and pediatric IBD compass.

17. Gupta K, Annapurna A, Verma P, Pal P, Supriya. Nurturing Bonds: A Holistic Guide to Breastfeeding Bliss. Hemakshee Publication. Sikar. 2024. ISBN: 978-81-969920-3-3.

Chapters of this book entitled **"Nurturing Bonds: A Holistic Guide to Breastfeeding Bliss"** particularly based on topics such as importance of breastfeeding to child and mothers, nurturing our future, infant food, promote breastfeeding, lactation and solemnization of the bond of motherhood, importance of breastfeeding- a holistic approach, nourishing empowerment, the significance of breastfeeding: a comprehensive comparison with infant formula feeding, breastfeeding in special circumstances, breastfeeding support in India, a mother's journey through breastfeeding, etc.

18. Gupta K, Das B, Deep EMS, Supriya, Singh S, Singhal AK. Handbook on Inflammatory Bowel Disease (Volume 2). Hemakshee Publication. Sikar. 2024. ISBN: 978-81-969920-1-9

This book titled **"Handbook on Inflammatory Bowel Disease (Volume 2)"** have chapters particularly based on topics such as classification of inflammatory bowel disease, IBD and its pathophysiology and morphology, role of nosodes in the treatment of inflammatory bowel disease ant its dietary management, curative treatment of inflammatory bowel disease by allopathy, the role of immunomodulators in inflammatory bowel disease, surgical treatment for IBD, role of residue in IBD, lactose intolerance and IBD: A comprehensive overview and IBD and mental health.

19. Gupta K, Supriya, Annapurna A, Sangeeta, Marwaha P. Nourishing Bonds: A Comprehensive Guide to Weaning. Hemakshee Publication. Sikar. 2024. ISBN: 978-81-971773-3-0.

The edited book volume is primarily intended to be a collection of selected short chapters written by research scholars, academicians, doctors and faculty members of their respective fields. Chapters of this book entitled **"Nourishing Bonds - A Comprehensive Guide to Weaning"** are particularly based on topics such as weaning, benefits to the baby through the process and stages of weaning, navigating the weaning journey: A holistic approach to infant nutrition, Weaning and complementary feeding: Feeding of an infant beyond 6 months age, guideline for weaning foods, issues related to weaning, **Challenges and opportunities of weaning, use of prebiotics and** probiotics in weaning food for infants, importance of finger foods in weaning, importance of weaning in infancy: A journey from dependency to diversity, Problems faced by the mother during breastfeeding and the child in weaning from breastfeeding etc.

20. Gupta K, Bajpai A, Verma P, Pal P, Singh T, Singh J. Skill Inculcation and Sustainable Community Development. Hemakshee Publication. Sikar. 2024. ISBN: 978-81-971773-7-8.

Chapters of this book particularly based on topics such as education for sustainable development, empowering sustainability: skill trainings for sustainable, skill building in India: institutes and government bodies at the helm, institutes and government bodies related to skill training, skill inculcation in ergonomics- promoting well being, safety and productivity, self help group and women empowerment, importance of skill development in textile sector, empowering Indian youth through food processing entrepreneurship trainings: an overview.

21. Gupta K, Tiwari T, Singh K,, Venkatappa KG, Chaturvedi B, Sangeeta. Empowering Future- Skill Inculcation and

Sustainable Communities. Hemakshee Publication. Sikar. 2024. ISBN: 978-81-971773-4-7.

Chapters of this book particularly based on topics such as life skills for students; empowering children with disabilities; skills to boost self confidence; personal skills; empowering communities: strategies for social, emotional and cognitive development; government programmes; the skill India mission; soft skills, emerging career opportunities in home science; vocational interest among academically backward rural children; refining your personality through skill development and role of upskilling, cross-skilling and reskilling.

22. Gupta K, Gunjan G, Vernekar GK, Mukharjee G, Sangeeta, Babu VS. Handbook on Inflammatory Bowel Disease (Volume 3). Hemakshee Publication. Sikar. 2024. ISBN: 978-81-978907-0-3

Chapters of this book were particularly based on topics such as dietary intervention in the management of irritable bowel syndrome, biological therapies in the treatment of inflammatory bowel disease, impact and risk factors of IBD on human health and life style, mental health implications of inflammatory bowel disease, irritable bowel disease and plant based diet, recipes to manage and cure inflammatory bowel diseases (IBD), evolving therapeutic strategies for inflammatory bowel disease: from conventional to cutting-edge approaches, IBD in women: fertility, pregnancy and beyond, current insights into the pathophysiology, histomorphology, and therapeutic advances in inflammatory bowel diseases.

23. Gupta K. Golden Guidelines for Optimizing Elderly Nutrition. Hemakshee Publication. Sikar. 2024. ISBN: 978-81-976151-3-9

Throughout this book, readers will find a wealth of information on topics such as nutrient requirements, the impact of aging on appetite and food choices, and the importance of personalized nutrition interventions. Additionally, practical insights into food-based interventions, fortification, and the development of nutrient-dense food products are provided to empower those caring for the elderly to make informed decisions that can enhance health outcomes.

24. Gupta K, supriya, Srivastava S, Saraswat M, Srivastava D, Sangeeta. Harmony in Diversity- Integrating Food, Textiles and Human Development in Communities. Hemakshee Publication. Sikar. 2024. ISBN: 978-81-978907-2-7.

In an era defined by rapid technological advances, shifting societal norms, and global health challenges, there is an urgent need to revisit the roots of community well-being. ***"Harmony in Diversity: Integrating Food, Textiles, and Human Development in Communities"*** seeks to explore the interdependent roles of food, textiles, and human development in shaping the fabric of society. This book represents a convergence of disciplines often perceived as separate, yet whose intersections hold untapped potential for fostering sustainable, healthy, and resilient communities.

Note: These books are available on publisher's website, Amazon and FlipKart